STUDENT WORKBOOK

by

Jude Franko, RN

TO ACCOMPANY

HOMEMAKER/HOME HEALTH AIDE

FOURTH EDITION

by
Helen Huber, BA
and
Audree Spatz, MEd, BSN, RN

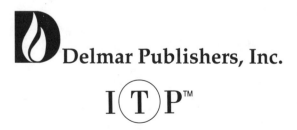

Delmar Publishers, Inc.

I(T)P™

NOTICE TO THE READER

For information, address

Delmar Publishers Inc.
3 Columbia Circle
Box 15015
Albany, New York 12212-5015

Printed in the United States of America
Published simultaneously in Canada
by Nelson Canada,
a division of The Thomson Corporation

3 4 5 6 7 8 9 10 XXX 00 99 98 97 96 95

ISBN: 0–8273–5273–5
Library of Congress Catalog Card Number: 92–40574

TABLE OF CONTENTS

INDEX OF COMPETENCY CHECKLISTS

INTRODUCTION TO THE STUDENT

Welcome to the world of home health care. This workbook lists the objectives for each unit of the text-book. Your instructor will provide information by way of handouts, video presentations, overheads, and class activities. They are ways in which you can become a more active learner. One type of an evaluation tool is a test or quiz. Another type may be active class participation in which you get to *plan* and *practice* in preparation for your final evaluations.

You can make the best of this workbook if you

    Read and study the unit you have been assigned
    Actively listen to the instructions given and the demonstrations provided
    Read and listen as the objectives are presented
    Are not afraid to ask questions

You have chosen an exciting and ever changing aspect of health care which requires a knowledgeable skilled individual to provide care for those who are in their own home and familiar surroundings. Best of luck to you — Enjoy.

Jude Franko

SECTION ONE
Overview of Units

SECTION 1   *Becoming a Home Health Aide*

UNIT 1   Home Health Services

OBJECTIVES

The student will be able to:

- Name three reasons why the trend toward home care has returned.
- Name the two services provided by the home health aide.
- Explain the difference between acute and chronic illness.
- Define DRGs.
- List two differences between Medicare and Medicaid.
- List one purpose of the CHAP program.
- Define OBRA.

UNIT SUMMARY

The homemaker/home health aide:

1. Needs knowledge and skill.
2. Needs to keep aware of changes in the home health care field.
3. Needs to be safe in giving proper skilled care.
4. Needs to be able to work with everyone on the home care team as well as family members.

TERMS TO DEFINE

1. acute illness_____
2. CHAP_____
3. chronic illness_____
4. developmentally disabled _____
5. home care aide_____
6. home health aide _____
7. homemaker_____
8. homemaker/home health aide _____
9. long-term care facilities_____
10. Medicaid _____
11. Medicare _____
12. OBRA_____
13. personal care worker _____

OBJECTIVES

The student will be able to:

- Define interpersonal relationships and interaction.
- Give an example of self-understanding.
- Identify the need for evaluation.
- State the difference between theory and practice.
- Give four examples of good personal hygiene.
- Identify five members of the health care team.

UNIT SUMMARY

The homemaker/home health aide:

1. Needs to be flexible and practice good work habits.
2. Needs to be sensitive to the various populations served.
3. Needs to present a professional appearance and good attitude for the client and family.

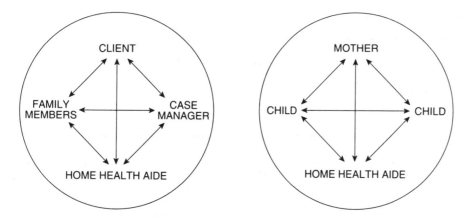

Figures 1 and 2   Home health aides interact with other care providers and family members.

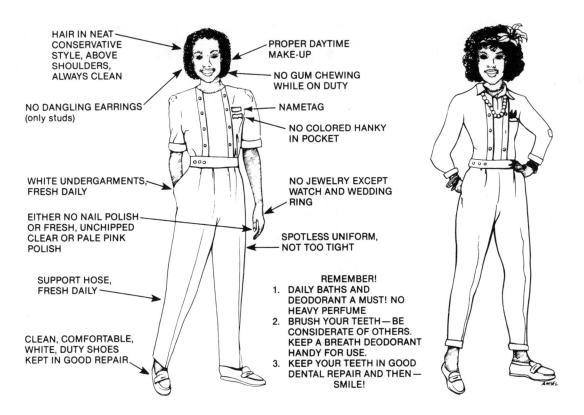

HAIR IN NEAT CONSERVATIVE STYLE, ABOVE SHOULDERS, ALWAYS CLEAN

PROPER DAYTIME MAKE-UP

NO GUM CHEWING WHILE ON DUTY

NO DANGLING EARRINGS (only studs)

NAMETAG

NO COLORED HANKY IN POCKET

WHITE UNDERGARMENTS, FRESH DAILY

NO JEWELRY EXCEPT WATCH AND WEDDING RING

EITHER NO NAIL POLISH OR FRESH, UNCHIPPED CLEAR OR PALE PINK POLISH

SPOTLESS UNIFORM, NOT TOO TIGHT

SUPPORT HOSE, FRESH DAILY

REMEMBER!
1. **DAILY BATHS AND DEODORANT A MUST! NO HEAVY PERFUME**
2. **BRUSH YOUR TEETH—BE CONSIDERATE OF OTHERS. KEEP A BREATH DEODORANT HANDY FOR USE.**
3. **KEEP YOUR TEETH IN GOOD DENTAL REPAIR AND THEN— SMILE!**

CLEAN, COMFORTABLE, WHITE, DUTY SHOES KEPT IN GOOD REPAIR

Figure 3 Contrast between proper and improper grooming for the homemaker/home health aide.

TERMS TO DEFINE

1. attitude _____

2. case manager _____

3. components _____

4. evaluation _____

5. hygiene _____

6. interaction _____

7. interpersonal relationships_____

8. LPN _____

9. offensive _____

10. oral hygiene _____

11. practice _____

12. procedure _____

13. RN _____

14. theory _____

OBJECTIVES

The student will be able to:

- Identify two career adjustments required of a home health aide.
- Name two client care responsibilities.
- Define ethics and identify two examples of ethical practice.
- Explain why accurate observation, reporting, and documentation are important tasks for the home health aide.
- Define the term "confidentiality."
- Explain what is meant by "liability" and give five examples of actions to avoid.
- List five "rights" of the client.
- List three "rights" of the home health aide.
- Define client abuse and list four types of client abuse.

UNIT SUMMARY

The homemaker/home health aide:

1. Needs to be aware of and adhere to ethical standards by respecting the client's rights.
2. Needs to maintain confidentiality.
3. Needs to accurately report and record the condition and behavior of the client in the home to the case manager.
4. Needs to be aware of the responsibility necessary to prevent injuries or accidents to the client or himself/herself.
5. Needs to be aware of the limitations of the duties performed by the home health aide.

TERMS TO DEFINE

1. abuse _____
2. career _____
3. confidentiality _____
4. documentation _____
5. ethics _____
6. flexible _____
7. liability _____
8. manipulation _____
9. negligence _____
10. client's rights _____

11. observation _____

11. reporting _____

12. time organization _____

OBJECTIVES

The student will be able to:

- Identify the sender-message-receiver process.
- Explain the difference between verbal and nonverbal communication.
- List four rules for improving aide/client communication.
- Identify two examples that apply rules of good communication.
- Identify characteristics of speech that affect communication.
- Give an example of a precise way to report an observation.

UNIT SUMMARY

The homemaker/home health aide:

1. Needs to communicate effectively, both verbally and nonverbally.
2. Needs to communicate clearly and accurately to the client, family members, visitors, and other members of the home care team.
3. Needs to be aware of the special terminology and abbreviations.
4. Needs to communicate to others with respect and dignity.

TERMS TO DEFINE

1. abbreviations _____
2. aphasia_____
3. body language _____
4. dyslexia _____
5. illiterate_____
6. listening_____
7. medical terminology _____
8. nonverbal communication _____
9. pitch _____
10. therapeutic _____
11. tone _____
12. verbal_____

UNIT 5 Understanding Differences: Individuals, Families, and Cultures

OBJECTIVES

The student will be able to:

- List three ways in which families may differ.
- Identify one way illness might affect a family.
- Discuss racial and religious prejudice.
- Identify what is meant by a family unit.
- Define environment and culture.
- List three main minority groups in the United States.
- Explain three different types of family units.
- Describe two typical differences between a family today and a family in the early part of this century.
- List two customs regarding health care that are different in a minority culture.

UNIT SUMMARY

The homemaker/home health aide:

1. Needs to be aware of the rules and standards in each family unit.
2. Needs to be aware of the "strange role" that the home health aide has as he or she works in a client's home.
3. Needs to take pride in the care provided to the client.

TERMS TO DEFINE

1. blended families_____
2. children with special needs_____
3. culture _____
4. divorce _____
5. environment _____
6. extended family _____
7. family unit_____
8. interracial family _____
9. life-style choices _____
10. living style _____
11. psychosocial _____
12. separation _____

13. single-parent families_____

14. two-career families _____

15. vegetarians _____

SECTION 2 *Basic Anatomy and Physiology*

UNIT 6 Functions and Disorders of the Body Systems

OBJECTIVES

The student will be able to:

- Identify one function of each body system.
- Name the five senses.
- Identify one disorder in each body system.
- Identify the relationship among cells, tissues, organs, and systems.
- Identify the difference between hereditary and environmental factors.
- List two factors that influence body development.

UNIT SUMMARY

The homemaker/home health aide:

1. Needs to know how the body functions during wellness.
2. Needs to know how the body is affected during illness or disease.
3. Needs to know how all body systems work together.
4. Needs to know how heredity and environment affect the health of the individual.

TERMS TO DEFINE

1. anemia _____
2. atherosclerosis _____
3. arthritis _____
4. auditory _____
5. bony prominences _____
6. contracture _____
7. cystitis _____
8. dermis _____
9. ducts _____
10. emphysema _____
11. epidermis _____
12. epilepsy _____
13. fracture _____
14. gangrene _____
15. hemiplegia _____
16. hemophiliac _____

17. hypertension _____

18. hypotension _____

19. impacted _____

20. incontinent _____

21. ligaments _____

22. otosclerosis _____

23. paraplegia _____

24. peristalsis _____

25. phlebitis _____

26. pressure areas _____

27. quadriplegia _____

28. sensory deficits _____

SECTION 3 *Understanding Human Development and Age-Related Health Problems*

UNIT 7   Infancy to Adolescence

OBJECTIVES

The student will be able to:

- Name five basic needs of the newborn infant.
- Identify three immunizations necessary for infants.
- List six disorders of the newborn.
- List four behavior patterns associated with abused children.
- List four conditions that can occur in an infant if the mother drinks alcohol during pregnancy.
- Recognize definitions for five of the key terms listed.
- Name two health problems that may affect adolescents.
- Identify changes that occur at puberty.

UNIT SUMMARY

The homemaker/home health aide:

1. Needs to know that life begins with the joining of a sperm and ovum.
2. Needs to know that as infants grow and develop, there are normal characteristics.
3. Needs to be aware of the needs of each age group to be able to meet those needs.

TERMS TO DEFINE

1. adolescence_____
2. bonding_____
3. cerebral palsy _____
4. cesarean section _____
5. child abuse _____
6. conception _____
7. cystic fibrosis_____
8. fetal alcohol syndrome _____
9. gestation period _____
10. immunity_____
11. low-birth-weight _____
12. premature _____

13. puberty _____

14. sibling rivalry _____

15. sudden infant death syndrome _____

OBJECTIVES

The student will be able to:

- List the causes of health problems in the early adult years.
- Describe the adjustments that often must be dealt with in the middle adult years.
- State why preventive health measures are important.
- Describe the changes that occur during the early and middle adult years in terms of family relationships.
- List two reasons a home health aide should encourage the client to exercise.
- List two activities a disabled client can become involved in outside of the home.

UNIT SUMMARY

The homemaker/home health aide:

1. Needs to know that changes occurring in early and middle adulthood require major adjustments.
2. Needs to be sensitive to people experiencing these changes.
3. Needs to be supportive and caring when helping individuals adjust to these changes.

TERMS TO DEFINE

1. early and middle adulthood _____
2. empty nest syndrome _____
3. mammogram _____
4. menopause _____
5. multiple sclerosis _____
6. Pap smear _____
7. preventive health measure _____
8. prognosis _____
9. rheumatoid arthritis _____
10. self-esteem _____
11. sigmoidoscopy _____

UNIT 9   Late Adulthood

OBJECTIVES

The student will be able to:

- Name some of the physical and emotional effects of the aging process.
- Identify the reasons for establishing regular schedules for elderly clients.
- Identify the effects of Alzheimer's disease.
- Describe the problems of persons confined to bed.
- Describe validation therapy.
- Describe the problems of clients who are nonambulatory.
- List five common chronic diseases of the elderly.

UNIT SUMMARY

The homemaker/home health aide:

1. Needs to be aware that as aging occurs, the body is slower to return to wellness after an injury or illness.
2. Needs to be aware of the changing and fragile degrees of psycho-social needs of the elderly client.
3. Needs to be aware of the normal changes during the later years of adulthood.

TERMS TO DEFINE

1. Alzheimer's disease _____
2. chronological _____
3. reality orientation _____
4. validation therapy _____

Observable

Hair: Thins and whitens

Vision: Declines; three out of five persons 75+ are affected to some degree, and more often in females than males.

Kidneys: Eventually lose up to 50 percent of their capacity to filter body wastes. This major system shows the greatest decline with age.

Heart:
1st—Between ages 20-90 the amount of blood pumped by the heart decreases 50 percent.
2nd—Muscle fibers contract more slowly.
3rd—Heart and blood vessels are more vulnerable to disease.

Bones: At 40+, the body no longer absorbs calcium efficiently, which contributes to fractures in more than 25 percent of all elderly women.

Joints: 1st—Begin to stiffen, particularly the hips and knees.
2nd—Compressed spinal discs shorten the body and cause a bent posture. Height loss of 1-3 inches is common.

Nervous System: 1st—Hardening of blood vessels create circulatory problems in the brain.
2nd—Aging reduces the speed with which the nervous system can process information or send signals for action.

Circulatory System: Failure in this system is the most common cause of death. Death from cardiovascular disease at age 75 is 150 times higher than at 35.

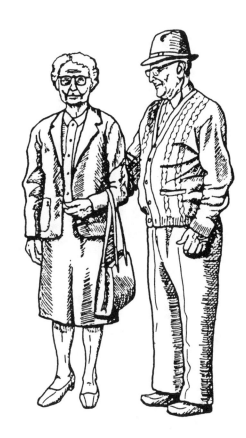

Nonobservable

Hearing:
1st—Ability to hear high pitches is more difficult.
2nd—Normal sound levels are more difficult to understand.

Skin:
1st—Fine lines around eyes and mouth.
2nd—Lines deepen into wrinkles.
3rd—Skin loses elasticity and smoothness.
4th—Spots of dark pigment.

Lungs:
1st—Between ages 30-75, the amount of air inhaled and exhaled drop by 45 percent.
2nd—Between ages 30-75, the amount of oxygen passing into the blood decreases about 50 percent.

Hormones:
1st—Decline in hormonal flow from the adrenal gland, located atop the kidney, lowers the ability of the elderly to respond to stress.
2nd—For women, menstruation ceases.

Immune System: This system becomes less efficient and therefore lowers the body's resistance to disease.

Muscles:
1st—There is a loss of muscle strength, which reduces coordination.
2nd—Lack of muscle tone causes a sagging of muscles.

Figure 4 Changes in the body over time. (Reprinted by permission from Zins, *Aging in America,* copyright 1987 by Delmar Publishers Inc.)

SECTION 4 *Promoting Health and Understanding Illness*

UNIT 10   Mental Health

OBJECTIVES

The student will be able to:

- Identify an example of a defense mechanism.
- Identify several common emotions.
- Identify how a physical response can result from an emotional reaction.
- Define psychology, mental health, and adjustments.
- Differentiate between external and internal stimuli.

UNIT SUMMARY

The homemaker/home health aide:

1. Needs to be aware of ways in which emotions affect behavior.
2. Needs to be aware that the body and the mind are able to adapt to changes.
3. Needs to be aware that all individuals respond with different emotions to different situations and that there are limits to acceptable behavior.

TERMS TO DEFINE

1. adjustment _____
2. anxiety _____
3. compensation _____
4. defense mechanism _____
5. denial _____
6. displacement _____
7. emotion _____
8. external stimulus _____
9. fantasizing _____
10. internal stimulus _____
11. mental illness _____
12. phobia _____
13. projection _____
14. psychology _____

15. rationalization _____

16. wellness _____

17. withdrawal_____

UNIT 11 Nutritional Guidelines

OBJECTIVES

The student will be able to:

- List the six food groups on the food guide pyramid.
- Identify the special diets used for at least five medical conditions.
- Name six things to keep in mind when planning and preparing meals.
- Name eight special diets that may be prescribed for your client, and describe the types of foods that are usually permitted for each.
- Identify the special diet a client with acquired immunodeficiency syndrome (AIDS) would require.

UNIT SUMMARY

The homemaker/home health aide:

1. Needs to be aware that food plays a major role in keeping the body in good working order.
2. Needs to be aware that proper nutrition must be practiced.
3. Needs to be aware of how to prepare and identify special diets as dictated by the plan of care.

TERMS TO DEFINE

1. bland diet _____
2. calorie-controlled diet _____
3. clear liquid diet _____
4. degenerative disease _____
5. diabetic diet _____
6. diuretic _____
7. empty calorie _____
8. food pyramid _____
9. full-liquid diet _____
10. high-bulk diet _____
11. low-residue diet _____
12. low-sodium diet _____
13. malnutrition _____
14. Meals on Wheels _____
15. nutrition _____
16. soft diet _____
17. vegetarian _____

UNIT 12   Principles of Safety and Body Mechanics

OBJECTIVES

The student will be able to:

- Identify five causes of accidents around the home.
- Name two conditions in aging which may contribute to the incidence of accidents.
- State the basic rules to follow in the event of a home fire.
- Define and demonstrate good body mechanics.
- List ten rules of good body mechanics.
- Briefly describe physical restraint.

UNIT SUMMARY

The homemaker/home health aide:

1. Needs to provide a safe environment for a client.
2. Needs to be aware of situations that can be unsafe in any area of the home.
3. Needs to know how to handle an emergency situation such as fire and falls, and what age groups are prone to accidents the most.
4. Needs to practice proper body mechanics to prevent self-injury or injury to a client.

TERMS TO DEFINE

1. body mechanics _____
2. cyanosis _____
3. evacuate_____
4. extinguish _____
5. hazard _____
6. immobilize _____
7. peripheral vision _____
8. transfer belt _____

UNIT 13 Understanding Illness

OBJECTIVES

The student will be able to:

- Identify the four cardinal signs and their normal values.
- Name three body sites where temperature is taken.
- Identify four signs that a client may be ill.
- Define rehabilitation.
- Explain the difference between a sign and a symptom.
- Describe the care given to the unconscious client.

UNIT SUMMARY

The homemaker/home health aide:

1. Needs to understand the emotional and physical aspects of illness or injury.
2. Needs to know how to measure and record the cardinal signs and report these to the case manager.
3. Needs to know how to give special care to the unconscious client.
4. Needs to be aware that the plan of care requires diversion as well as recreation and rehabilitation.

TERMS TO DEFINE

1. acute _____
2. apnea _____
3. blood pressure _____
4. bradycardia _____
5. cardinal signs _____
6. Cheyne-Stokes _____
7. chronic _____
8. contracture _____
9. diastolic _____
10. dyspnea _____
11. pulse _____
12. rales _____
13. range of motion exercises _____
14. rehabilitation _____
15. respiration _____

16. sign _____

17. sphygmomanometer _____

18. symptoms _____

19. systolic _____

20. tachycardia _____

CARE REQUIRED	FREQUENCY	WHAT TO DO
Mouth care	Every 2 hours	Wipe tongue, lips, gums, and teeth with gauze pad or cotton swab moistened with water or mouthwash. Lubricate and moisten mouth tissues with glycerin or vegetable oil. Wipe away saliva as it dribbles from mouth.
	When client vomits	Turn client to side at first sign of vomiting. Catch vomitus in a bowl or basin held to the side of the mouth. Wipe mouth with gauze pads or clean damp cloth.
Eye care	Wipe clean in AM and PM	Cover eyelids with soft cloth moistened in pre-boiled water. (Prevents eye cavity from becoming dry, since eyes may not close or blink.)
Repositioning	At least every 2 hours	Turn from back to side, and side to front, etc. (This prevents pressure sores from forming.)
Range of Motion (ROM) exercises	As ordered by doctor	Exercise all client's body parts if permitted. (Keeps blood circulating, prevents contractures, and prevents loss of motion in joints.)
Body massage with lotion	At least daily	Rub skin firmly but gently. Rub in a circular motion around bony prominences.
Care of bowel and bladder drainage	At least every hour	Check perineal area and bed linens to see if they are clean and dry. If client has not voided for 8 hours, report it to the supervisor. If client has not had bowel movement for 2 days, report it to the supervisor.
Accident prevention	At all times	Put up guard rails or place chairs beside bed to prevent falls. Observe for signs of vomiting and keep saliva wiped away; client may choke or inhale fluids into the lungs. Keep blankets and pillows away from the client's nose and mouth to avoid smothering.
Easy access to client	At all times	Safety and ease of working with client. Place the bed away from the wall so both sides of the bed are accessible.
Room ventilation	Open windows or vent daily	Keep temperature between 66°–70°, keep drafts from client. Open windows or vents to circulate air.
Tender Loving Care (TLC)	At all times	Talk to the client as if the client were conscious. Client may be able to hear and understand. (Communication gives client link with reality.) Use gentle touch often. If time allows, hold the client's hands and run fingers across forehead.

Figure 5   Care required on some clients' plan of care.

OBJECTIVES

The student will be able to:

- Name three different types of microorganisms.
- Identify three universal precaution techniques.
- Give three examples of ways germs can spread from one person to another.
- Give three examples of situations requiring universal precautions.
- Name the single most effective precaution to prevent spread of infections.
- List five times when aides must wash their hands.

UNIT SUMMARY

The homemaker/home health aide:

1. Needs to be aware of the microorganisms that cause disease and how to prevent these microorganisms from spreading.
2. Needs to be aware of the body's natural defenses against disease and help the client to maintain these defenses.

TERMS TO DEFINE

1. asepsis _____
2. bacteria _____
3. contagious _____
4. contaminated _____
5. disinfected _____
6. fungi _____
7. germs _____
8. incubation period _____
9. infection control _____
10. isolation _____
11. microorganisms _____
12. pathogens _____
13. protozoa _____
14. rickettsiae _____
15. sterile _____
16. universal precautions _____
17. virus _____

UNIT 15   Caring for the Client with an Infectious Disease

OBJECTIVES

The student will be able to:

- Recognize, define, and use key terms appropriately.
- List two contagious/infectious diseases.
- Explain the signs and symptoms and nursing care for a client with tuberculosis.
- Explain the signs and symptoms and nursing care for a client with hepatitis B.
- Recognize and discuss ethical problems regarding the client with acquired immunodeficiency syndrome (AIDS).
- Describe the common signs and symptoms of AIDS.
- Discuss the emotional needs of an AIDS client.
- List six rules to follow when caring for a client with an infectious disease.
- List six precautions or guidelines to follow when caring for an AIDS client.

UNIT SUMMARY

The homemaker/home health aide:

1. Needs to be aware that tuberculosis is increasing in the United States.
2. Needs to be aware that hepatitis B can be prevented by vaccination.
3. Needs to be aware of the signs and symptoms of AIDS and how to physically and emotionally care for a client with AIDS.

TERMS TO DEFINE

1. AIDS_____

2. AZT _____

3. contagious_____

4. empathy_____

5. hepatitis A_____

6. hepatitis B_____

7. HIV _____

8. homosexual _____

9. immune deficiency _____

10. infection _____

11. infectious disease _____

12. invasion _____

13. jaundice_____

14. tuberculosis _____

SAMPLE CARE PLAN FOR CLIENT WITH AIDS

SIGN/SYMPTOM	CARE TO PROVIDE	PURPOSE
Weakness/tiredness	High calorie diet with inbetween meal high protein snacks.	To provide protein nutrition and to slow muscle deterioration.
Fever	Sponge baths, give additional fluids by mouth; cover with blankets during chill periods.	To lower the temperature and to prevent complications. To get client comfortable.
Night sweats	Sponge baths, frequent linen changes, give additional fluids to avoid dehydration.	To provide comfort and to return skin to normal condition.
Cough	Observe and record patterns and changes and report findings. Offer cough medicine if prescribed. Gloves required when working.	To make the client comfortable and to obtain relief from strain.
Dyspnea	Note patterns and changes—record and report. Calm client and avoid exertion by client and help with breathing exercises.	To provide breath control and relaxation.
Skin lesions	Keep client from scratching—be sure nails are properly cut by nurse—wear gloves when working with client with lesions and wash hands carefully after contact with client.	To prevent infections.
Dry hair and hair loss	Avoid too frequent shampooing—use mild shampoo containing no alcohol. Use hair conditioner.	To prevent further hair loss and scalp irritation.
Mouth lesions	Provide saline or anesthetic mouthwashes; brush teeth gently. Check to be sure client can swallow without difficulty—observe, record, and report to supervisor. Avoid spicy, acid foods and carbonated beverages. Gloves are required when giving mouth care.	To provide infection control, client comfort, and adequate nutrition.

Figure 6   Sample care plan for client with AIDS.

SIGN/SYMPTOM	CARE TO PROVIDE	PURPOSE
Diarrhea	Encourage fluid intake; change linens as needed; apply brief if required; observe, record, and report; gloves required.	To maintain nutrition and fluid balance. To prevent pressure sore formation.
Impaired Immune System (when client picks up any infection around)	Give daily shower or bath; both client and HHC wash hands frequently; request nurse to apply sterile dressings as needed with gloves; do not allow visitors who have infections, such as colds; do not come to give client care if you are suffering from any infection.	To prevent infection and to assist in client protection.
Unstable emotional responses	Be aware of client's feelings as well as your own. Be honest with client and accept him as a person, not as an AIDS victim. Offer emotional support, kindness. Communicate by touching client's hand, pat on back, etc.	To create an atmosphere of mutual trust.

THE FOLLOWING RULES ARE DESIGNED TO PREVENT TRANSMISSION OF THE INFECTION:
1. Wear a gown if there is a possibility of soiling your clothing with blood or body secretions of client.
2. Wear gloves when touching blood or body secretions.
3. Wash hands before and after client contact and immediately if they are potentially contaminated with blood or body secretions.
4. Discard articles contaminated with blood or body secretions and secure in plastic bag.
5. IF YOU HAVE AN OPEN CUT OR WOUND DO NOT CONTAMINATE THE WOUND WITH CLIENT'S BODY SECRETIONS.
6. Follow any additional instructions by your supervisor or case manager.

Figure 6 *(Continued)*   Sample care plan for client with AIDS.

| DISEASE | COMMON COMMUNICABLE DISEASES | | |
	HOW IT ENTERS BODY	HOW IT LEAVES BODY	HOW IT IS TRANSFERRED
Pneumonia	mouth to lungs	sputum, nasal discharge	direct contact, articles used by and around patient, hands
Influenza	mouth/nose to lungs	as above	as above
Tuberculosis	mouth/lungs/ intestines/lymph system	sputum, lesions, feces	kissing, coughing, sputum, soiled dressings, hands
Poliomyelitis	mouth/nose	nasal and throat discharges	direct contact hands
Measles(rubella)	mouth/nose	nasal/throat discharges	direct contact, articles used by and around patients, hands
Gonorrhea	mucous membrane	body discharges, lesions	sexual intercourse, towels, linens, toilets, hands
Syphilis	blood and tissues through skin breaks	infected tissues, lesions placenta to fetus	direct contact, kissing, sexual intercourse
AIDS	mucous membrane, blood, any discharge containing blood	placenta to fetus, transfusion, body discharges, blood	sexual intercourse (anal, oral, and vaginal), needles and syringes
Hepatitis A	mouth/intestine	feces	direct contact, contaminated water, contaminated food
Hepatitis B	blood contact	blood	blood transfusion, contaminated needles or instrument

Figure 7 Common communicable diseases.

SECTION 5 *Caring for Clients with Acute and Chronic Disorders*

UNIT 16   Caring for Clients with Diabetes

OBJECTIVES

The student will be able to:

- Name four signs and symptoms of diabetes.
- List four types of diabetes.
- Name three ways of controlling diabetes.
- Describe the procedure for testing blood sugar with the use of a glucometer.
- Name three long-term complications of diabetes.
- List signs and symptoms for insulin shock and diabetic coma and the immediate care for each.
- Explain special foot care given to the diabetic client.
- Describe special techniques used in caring for a client who has vision impairment.

UNIT SUMMARY

The homemaker/home health aide:

1. Needs to be aware that diabetes is treated with exercise, diet, and drug therapy.
2. Needs to be aware that many people may have signs and symptoms of diabetes and not be aware of it.
3. Needs to be aware that major complications of diabetes can develop.
4. Needs to be aware that preventive health care can save the client needless pain and suffering.

TERMS TO DEFINE

1. blood lancet _____
2. cyanotic _____
3. diabetes _____
4. gangrene _____
5. gestational _____
6. glucometer _____
7. glucose _____
8. hormone _____
9. insulin _____
10. hyperglycemia _____
11. hypoglycemic _____
12. subcutaneously _____

LONG-TERM DISORDERS	CAUSE	SYMPTOMS	TREATMENT	AIDE'S CARE
Blindness	Cataracts, glaucoma, hemorrhage	Partial or total loss of sight, client drops items, stumbles or falls; develops tunnel vision	Surgery can remove cataracts; lost sight from glaucoma cannot be restored; save what sight remains	Assist in activities of daily living
Gas gangrene	Poor circulation; skin breakdown; invasion of tissue by bacteria	Heat in area, skin reddened, formation of ulcers that don't clear up; foul odor and spread of infection and tissue destruction	Medication under doctor's order; may require amputation of limb	Assist with dressing changes and rehabilitation
Kidney disease	Too much sugar free in urine; filtering system works inefficiently	Frequency, pain, burning while voiding; retention of urine may occur	Diet modification and medication	Observe and record Intake/Output; note color and compostion of urine
Vascular disease and nerve degeneration	High sugar level; poor fat metabolism; poor tissue repair; poor circulation	Open lesions form on skin tissue as vascular degeneration occurs; nervous system functions at decreased level—sight, sound, taste, touch, smell may be affected	Bedrest, moist heat/dressings; diet and medication	Give proper foot care. Assist in activities of daily living

Figure 8   Complications of diabetes.

UNIT 17 Caring for Clients with Circulatory Disorders

OBJECTIVES

The student will be able to:

- Identify symptoms of four heart conditions.
- Describe care given for clients with heart conditions.
- Explain the effect nitroglycerin has on the blood vessels.
- Give two other names for a CVA.
- List six risk factors for heart attacks and strokes.
- List three signs a client might display if suffering from a heart attack.
- List four warning signs of stroke.
- List three causes of stroke.
- List two types of aphasia.
- List three physical defects a client may have following a stroke.
- Explain the role of the aide in assisting a client recovering from a stroke.

UNIT SUMMARY

The homemaker/home health aide:

1. Needs to be aware of the basic heart conditions.
2. Needs to be aware of a change for the worse in the client's condition and contact help.
3. Needs to be aware also that diet, exercise, rest periods, and medication are special cares needed by a client with disorders of the heart and circulatory system.

TERMS TO DEFINE

1. aneurysm_____
2. angina pectoris_____
3. anticoagulants _____
4. aphasia_____
5. arteriogram_____
6. arteriosclerosis _____
7. artery_____
8. atherosclerosis _____
9. cardiac arrest _____
10. catheterization _____
11. cerebral hemorrhage_____
12. cerebral vascular accident (CVA)_____
13. collateral circulation _____

14. congestive heart failure _____

15. edema _____

16. embolus _____

17. expressive aphasia _____

18. ischemia _____

19. myocardial infarction _____

20. myocardium _____

21. nitroglycerin _____

22. occupational therapist _____

23. receptive aphasia _____

24. spasticity _____

25. sublingually _____

26. thrombus _____

27. transient ischemic attack (TIA) _____

UNIT 18   Caring for Clients with Arthritis

OBJECTIVES

The student will be able to:

- Describe the care given to clients with arthritis.
- Define the terms relating to arthritis.
- Discuss the exercises related to arthritis.
- Define osteoarthritis, rheumatoid arthritis, and gout.
- List two types of diets that may be prescribed for clients with arthritis.
- List three side effects of steroids.
- List two goals of an exercise program for a client with arthritis.
- Name two joints that can be replaced by surgery.

UNIT SUMMARY

The homemaker/home health aide:

1. Needs to be aware that clients with arthritis have limited activities on some days and that exercise needs to be adjusted.
2. Needs to be aware that activity and exercise as well as good nutrition and pain control are essential to the client with arthritis.

TERMS TO DEFINE

1. arthritis _____

2. degenerative _____

3. gout _____

4. joint inflammation _____

5. osteoarthritis _____

6. rheumatism _____

7. rheumatoid _____

8. steroids _____

9. tophi _____

OBJECTIVES

The student will be able to:

- Identify three diagnostic tests for cancer.
- Identify six surgical procedures used in cancer treatment.
- List seven warning signs of cancer.
- Define metastasis, benign tumor, remission, and malignant.
- Name three types of treatment for cancer.
- Describe the care given to a client with cancer.
- List two precautions for an aide to take when caring for a client who is on chemotherapy.

UNIT SUMMARY

The homemaker/home health aide:

1. Needs to be aware that clients are treated with surgery, radiation, and chemotherapy, and that special care is required.
2. Needs to try to make the client as comfortable and cheerful as possible.
3. Needs to be aware of the emotional stress suffered by the client and the family.

TERMS TO DEFINE

1. articulates _____
2. benign _____
3. biopsy_____
4. cancer _____
5. carcinogen _____
6. chemotherapy_____
7. colostomy _____
8. expectorate _____
9. hysterectomy_____
10. ileostomy_____
11. irrigation_____
12. laryngectomy _____
13. larynx_____
14. lobectomy _____
15. malignant _____

16. mammogram _____

17. mastectomy _____

18. metastasis _____

19. metastasize _____

20. pneumonectomy _____

21. remission _____

22. stoma _____

23. trachea_____

24. tracheostomy _____

OBJECTIVES

The student will be able to:

- Identify some cultural influences surrounding practices related to death.
- Identify the five stages of dying as described by Dr. Kübler-Ross.
- Identify the home health aide's responsibilities when the client dies.
- Identify ways in which a person may react to the death of a family member or friend.
- Become familiar with the needs of a dying client.
- Explain the Patient Self-Determination Act.
- Define the purpose of hospice programs.
- Explain the importance of grief.

UNIT SUMMARY

The homemaker/home health aide:

1. Needs to be aware of the stages of loss and death.
2. Needs to be aware of the cultural influences that have an effect on the concept of death and dying.
3. Needs to keep the client as comfortable as possible and assist the family as needed when death occurs.

TERMS TO DEFINE

1. advanced directives _____
2. durable power of attorney _____
3. embalming _____
4. grieve _____
5. hospice _____
6. living will _____
7. postmortem _____
8. terminally _____

UNIT 21   Principles of Household Management

OBJECTIVES

The student will be able to:

- List at least four tips used to plan and organize tasks.
- Explain how to care for major home appliances.
- State some ways to combine client care and household tasks.

UNIT SUMMARY

The homemaker/home health aide:

1. Needs to be aware that doing household tasks is an important part of the duties required by the client.
2. Needs to be able to operate household equipment and appliances to provide a clean and safe environment.

TERMS TO DEFINE

1. instinct _____

2. myth _____

GENERAL HOUSEHOLD SAFETY CHECKLIST	
1. Are stairs, halls, and exits free from clutter?	_____
2. Are throw rugs eliminated or fastened down?	_____
3. Are electrical cords in good condition?	_____
4. Is furniture arranged to allow free movement in heavy traffic areas? (Don't re-arrange furniture without permission.)	_____
5. Is storage space easy to reach in areas where often-used items are stored?	_____
6. Are pot handles turned toward the back of the stove?	_____
7. Are grease and liquids wiped up immediately when spilled?	_____
8. Are cleaning fluids, polishes, bleaches, detergents, and all poisons stored separately and clearly marked?	_____
9. Is bath or shower temperature checked with the hand before showering or bathing?	_____
10. Are medicines clearly labeled when they are for external use only?	_____
11. Are shoes kept well-tied and worn for household activities instead of bedroom slippers?	_____
12. Are hazardous tools and firearms kept stored away safely?	_____

Figure 9   General household safety checklist.

OBJECTIVES

The student will be able to:

- Name three factors that determine the aide's cleaning plan.
- List five cleaning tasks done daily.
- List five cleaning tasks done weekly.
- List five cleaning tasks done only periodically.
- Describe the correct method for separating and disposing of garbage.
- Identify at least four steps used in cleaning a kitchen.
- Identify daily bathroom care that family members should perform.
- Identify two bathroom cleaning tasks the aide does daily.

UNIT SUMMARY

The homemaker/home health aide:

1. Needs to be aware that certain household tasks are done on a daily, weekly, or monthly basis.
2. Needs to develop an organized cleaning schedule that prevents task overload for the home health aide and at the same time meets the family and client needs.

TERMS TO DEFINE

1. mildew _____
2. pathogens _____
3. sanitary _____

OBJECTIVES

The student will be able to:

- List four guidelines for planning menus.
- State eight guidelines for buying foods.
- List four guidelines for storing food.
- Name five guidelines for preparing meals.

UNIT SUMMARY

The homemaker/home health aide:

1. Needs to be aware that marketing and meal preparation are important responsibilities.
2. Needs to be aware of specific guidelines provided by a dietitian when preparing meals.
3. Needs to be aware of budget limits when marketing.
4. Needs to store cooked and uncooked food properly.

CHECK SHEET ON COOKING HAZARDS	
1. Always wash hands thoroughly before handling food.	_____
2. Keep pot and pan handles positioned toward back of stove.	_____
3. Avoid clothing with long flowing sleeves that may easily catch on pot handles and/or cause burns.	_____
4. Clean up spills on floors immediately to prevent falling.	_____
5. Avoid broken or chipped cooking utensils or serving pieces.	_____
6. Turn off the range and oven when not in use.	_____
7. Check electric cords on appliances periodically for worn places.	_____
8. Avoid overloading electric outlets. Unplug appliances that are not in use.	_____
9. Dry hands before using electrical appliances.	_____
10. Encourage family to have gas ranges periodically checked by gas company.	_____
11. Store knives carefully.	_____
12. If possible, keep a box of baking soda near the stove to	

Figure 10   Check sheet on cooking hazards.

TERMS TO DEFINE

1. bulk _____

2. convenience foods _____

3. delicatessen _____

4. fermented _____

5. perishable _____

6. produce _____

7. staple items _____

UNIT 24   Laundry Duties

OBJECTIVES

The student will be able to:

- Identify two ways to sort clothes for washing.
- Identify the best time to perform mending.
- Identify several methods for removing stains.
- Explain how to wash clothing and bed linens from a client with an infectious disease.

UNIT SUMMARY

The homemaker/home health aide:

1. Needs to follow instructions on washing machine and dryer before doing laundry.
2. Needs to sort unlaundered clothes and bedding in a proper manner.
3. Needs to be aware of special laundering needs of certain articles of clothing.

TERMS TO DEFINE

1. agitator _____
2. permanent press _____
3. polyester fabrics _____

SECTION 7 *Health Care Services*

UNIT 25   Introduction to Client Care Procedures

OBJECTIVES

The student will be able to:

- List the rules for carrying out client care procedures.
- Describe how to provide privacy for the client during procedures.
- State when the aide's hands should be washed.
- Explain why it is necessary to give an explanation to the client before doing any procedure.
- Recognize those procedures which you, as a home health aide, are not permitted to do because of state mandated guidelines or agency's policies.

UNIT SUMMARY

The homemaker/home health aide:

1. Needs to gain cooperation and participation of a client.
2. Needs to let the client actively assist as much as possible.
3. Needs to always maintain safety and privacy and to explain what is being done.
4. Needs to be as efficient and safe as possible when helping someone who is totally dependent.
5. Needs to recognize limitations because of state, federal, or agency policies.

UNIT 26 Infection Control and Universal Precautions

OBJECTIVES

The student will be able to:

- Demonstrate clear ability to perform all the procedures.
- Explain the purpose of each procedure.
- State when the procedures should and should not be done.
- Identify precautions to be taken for each procedure.

UNIT SUMMARY

The homemaker/home health aide:

1. Needs to maintain a clean environment by means of hand washing and using personal protective equipment.

OBJECTIVES

The student will be able to:

- Demonstrate clear ability to perform all procedures.
- Explain the purpose of each procedure.
- Identify precautions to be taken for each procedure.
- Use proper body mechanics for both client and aide doing each procedure.
- Move the client without injury to either client or aide.
- Identify altered body alignment.
- Increase client independence and aid rehabilitation.

UNIT SUMMARY

The homemaker/home health aide:

1. Needs to be aware of the necessity to be able to lift, move, position, exercise, transfer, and assist a client.

OBJECTIVES

The student will be able to:

- Demonstrate clear ability to perform all procedures.
- Explain the purpose of each procedure.
- State when the procedures should and should not be done.
- Be aware of precautions to take with each procedure.
- Demonstrate the use of universal precautions when doing each procedure.

UNIT SUMMARY

The homemaker/home health aide:

1. Needs to be aware of the importance of giving and/or assisting with bathing.
2. Needs to be aware of the necessity for special skin care.

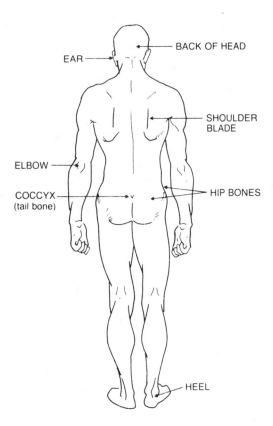

Figure 11   Common sites for pressure sores.

OBJECTIVES

The student will be able to:

- Demonstrate clear ability to perform all procedures.
- Explain the purpose of each procedure.
- State when the procedures should and should not be done.
- Be aware of precautions to take with each procedure.
- Demonstrate the use of universal precautions when handling body substances.

UNIT SUMMARY

The homemaker/home health aide:

1. Needs to be able to carry out routine daily care as stated in the plan of care.

OBJECTIVES

The student will be able to:

- Demonstrate clear ability to perform all procedures.
- Explain the purpose of each procedure.
- Calculate, record, and report results of all procedures.
- Encourage client to do as much as possible with remaining abilities.
- Be aware of precautions to take with every procedure.

UNIT SUMMARY

The homemaker/home health aide:

1. Needs to be able to carry out the feeding and toileting needs of the client.

OBJECTIVES

The student will be able to:

- Demonstrate clear ability to perform all the procedures.
- Explain the purpose of each procedure.
- Use universal precautions when handling body substances.
- Recognize abnormal conditions.
- Report and record observations.

UNIT SUMMARY

The homemaker/home health aide:

1. Needs to be able to safely and accurately record urinary output and safely and effectively handle urinary drainage equipment.

OBJECTIVES

The student will be able to:

- Demonstrate clear ability to perform all the procedures.
- Explain the purpose of each procedure.
- State when the procedures should and should not be done.
- Identify precautions to be taken for each procedure.
- Recognize abnormal readings.
- Record vital signs properly.

UNIT SUMMARY

The homemaker/home health aide:

1. Needs to be aware of the normal ranges of all the cardinal signs.
2. Needs to be able to accurately check the cardinal signs.

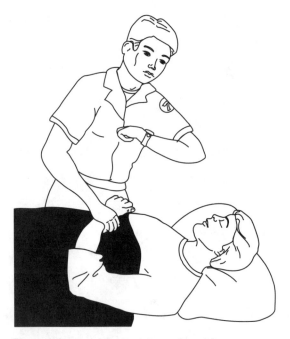

Figure 12   In this position, the aide can count the pulse and then see and feel the client breathing while counting respirations.

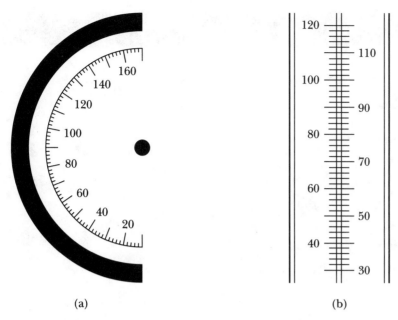

(a)   (b)

Figure 13 Two types of blood pressure devices.

OBJECTIVES

The student will be able to:

- Demonstrate clear ability to perform all procedures.
- Explain the purpose of each procedure.
- State when the procedures should and should not be done.
- Identify precautions to be taken for each procedure.
- Recognize signs of client discomfort.
- Follow all rules of client safety when doing the procedures.

UNIT SUMMARY

The homemaker/home health aide:

1. Needs to be aware of the benefits ofapplying hot and cold applications.
2. Needs to recognize the dangers of hot or cold applications.

UNIT 34 Rectal Care

OBJECTIVES

The student will be able to:

- Demonstrate clear ability to perform all the procedures.
- Explain the purpose of each procedure.
- State when the procedures should and should not be done.
- Demonstrate universal precautions when doing the procedures.
- Record and report results of all procedures.

UNIT SUMMARY

The homemaker/home health aide:

1. Needs to be aware of the reasons for giving suppositories or enemas.
2. Needs to be aware that putting on an adult brief requires skill and sensitivity.

OBJECTIVES

The student will be able to:

- Demonstrate clear ability to perform all procedures.
- Explain the purpose of each procedure.
- State when the procedures should and should not be done.
- Be aware of precautions to take with each procedure.
- Report and record unusual different signs and symptoms that you observe.

UNIT SUMMARY

The homemaker/home health aide:

1. Needs to be aware of the limitations for doing special treatments.

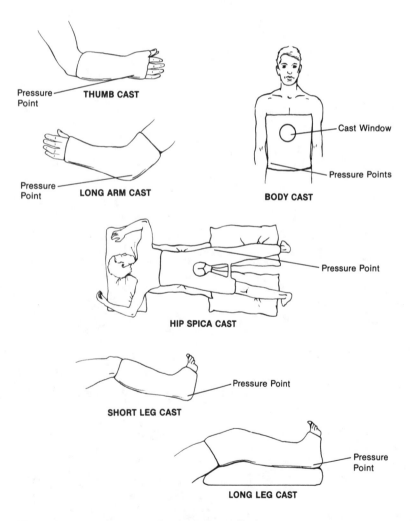

Figure 14   Casts that are frequently applied.

OBJECTIVES

The student will be able to:

- Demonstrate clear ability to perform all procedures.
- Explain the purpose of each procedure.
- State when the procedures should and should not be done.
- Identify precautions to be taken with each procedure.

UNIT SUMMARY

The homemaker/home health aide:

1. Needs to be aware of the needs of the infant and mother when performing care.

SECTION 8 *Employment*

UNIT 37 Job-seeking Skills

OBJECTIVES

The student will be able to:

- Accurately fill out an employment application.
- Prepare a resume and/or personal information sheet.
- Present yourself in a professional manner to a prospective employer during an interview.
- Select an agency to apply for employment.

UNIT SUMMARY

The homemaker/home health aide:

1. Needs to provide a prospective employer with a complete application form and conduct himself or herself during the interview with pride and self-assurance.

TERMS TO DEFINE

1. diagnosis related groups _____

2. infraction _____

3. misconduct _____

4. personal reference _____

5. registry service _____

APPLICATION FOR EMPLOYMENT

We are an equal opportunity employer. Federal and state laws prohibit discrimination in employment practices based on race, color, religion, sex, age, handicap, disability, or national origin. No question on this application is asked for the purpose of limiting or excluding any applicant's consideration for employment because of his or her race, color, religion, sex, age, handicap, disability, or national origin.

Name: Last	First	Middle	Social Security No.	Telephone No.

Address: Street	City	State	Zip Code	Licensed Nurses Only	
				Mass. Reg. No.	Date Granted:

If your records may be under a name other than indicated above, please specify:	Last Renewal:	Expiration Date:

Are you a citizen of the United States? ☐ yes ☐ no	If you are not a U.S. Citizen, do you have the legal right to remain permanently in the United States? ☐ yes ☐ no	Explain
Are you between the ages of 18 and 70? ☐ yes ☐ no	Do you know of any fact that would limit or impair your ability to perform the functions of the job you are applying for? ☐ yes ☐ no	Describe

Date of last Physical Examination:	Family Physician:	I authorize my doctor to release to you the results of my pre-employment and subsequent medical examinations, and to discuss those results with you. ☐ yes ☐ no

Position desired:	Hours desired:	Salary expected:

Specialized training or experience not shown on other side of form:

Where now employed?	Reason for desiring change:

Have you ever pleaded guilty or been convicted of a felony? ☐ yes ☐ no	If yes to either, please explain:

or a misdemeanor other than a first conviction for drunkenness, simple assault, speeding, minor ☐ yes traffic violations, affray, or disturbance of the peace ☐ no within the past 5 years?

In case of emergency notify	name	relationship
	address	telephone

*I authorize the schools, employers, and individuals listed in this application to release any information regarding my previous employment, character, general reputation and personal characteristics. ☐ yes ☐ no

I certify that the statements I have made in this application are true and hereby grant the employer permission to verify the accuracy and completeness of this information and to investigate all references and educational records. I understand that any false or misleading statements made by me on this application or in conjunction with my physical examination will be sufficient cause for the rejection of this application or for immediate dismissal if such false or misleading information is discovered after my employment. If I am accepted for employment, I agree to abide by the rules and regulations of the employer.

Signed ————————————————————

Date ————————————————————

Figure 15   Sample application form.

SECTION TWO
Application Exercises

1. The homemaker/home health aide works under the supervision of a:

    a. physician

    b. case manager

    c. client

    d. health care agency

2. The homemaker/home health aide's duties may include:

    a. revising the care plan

    b. teaching indirectly

    c. checking the blood pressure

    d. cutting a diabetic's toenails

3. Susie Que, a homemaker/home health aide, wakes up with a cold, sore throat, cough, and a temperature of 101°F on a day she is assigned to care for a client. What should Susie do?

    a. telephone the agency as soon as possible

    b. take a cold tablet and go to work as usual

    c. go to work and wear a mask when she is with the client

    d. go to work and call the agency from the client's home

4. Nonverbal communication skills would include:

    a. frowning

    b. standing with your arms crossed

    c. smiling

    d. all of the above

The next five questions refer to the following situation:

You are assigned to care for Etta, a 79-year-old-widow who lives alone. Etta was independent until she fell and broke her hip. Etta needs help bathing, making meals, cleaning her house, and paying bills.

5. On your first day, Etta tries to get up and walk with a walker before she is supposed to. Etta says, "I hate having to depend on someone else all the time." To show Etta that you understand her feelings, what should you say?

    a. "You shouldn't feel that way. That's what I'm here for."

    b. "You make me unhappy when you talk like that."

    c. "It's hard to have someone help you when you're used to doing it yourself."

    d. "You should like being taken care of."

6. Etta is hard of hearing. In order to communicate most effectively with her, you should:

    a. yell loudly into her good ear

    b. speak clearly, looking directly at Etta

    c. try to speak very slowly

    d. use a high-pitched voice

7. The reaction to illness that Etta is showing is most likely:

    a. anger

    b. depression

    c. dependence

    d. overdependence

8. Your long-term goal with Etta would be to:

    a. promote her self-care and independence

    b. promote bedrest as much as possible so she does not fall again

    c. respect her privacy

    d. have her placed in a nursing home

9. One day, while caring for Etta, you notice a reddened area on her hip. In addition to reporting it to the case manager, you should:

    a. rub the client's back thoroughly and position the client so no pressure is on the area

    b. rub the client's back but do not rub the lower part of the back near the red area

    c. omit the backrub and apply corn-starch to the red area

    d. omit the backrub and place a dressing over the red area

10. An infant's pulse is normally

    a. 180

    b. 90

    c. 130

    d. 72

11. A 2-year-old who says "no" to everything you say is most likely:

    a. slow at learning

    b. showing regression

    c. going to have problems later in life

    d. trying to assert independence

12. Rubbing the lower back of a bedridden client at frequent intervals helps to prevent the development of bed sores in this area chiefly by:

    a. softening the skin

    b. increasing the thickness of the skin and underlying tissue

    c. improving the circulation to the part

    d. keeping the skin cool

13. In addition to washing the hands and face, a partial bath generally includes washing the:

   a. chest and legs

   b. arms and legs

   c. feet, abdomen, and chest

   d. armpits, back, and genitals

14. A client is to have a record kept of his/her fluid intake. One day, while you are present, the client drinks the following fluids: ¾ glass milk, ⅔ cup tea, and ⅓ bowl soup. The glass holds 8 ounces of fluid, or 240 cc; the cup and bowl each hold 6 ounces, or 180 cc each (remember: 30 cc = 1 ounce). The client's total fluid intake is:

   a. 12 ounces

   b. 16 ounces

   c. 18 ounces

   d. 20 ounces

15. Mr. C. has had a resting pulse of 84–92 for the last 3 days. When you take it today, it is 110 resting. What should you do?

   a. Record the pulse as usual

   b. notify the case manager immediately

   c. tell the client to walk around inside the house

   d. place a warm cloth on the client's forehead

16. While you are working with a client who is terminally ill, the client states, "If only I could live long enough to see my children grow up, I wouldn't mind being sick." This client is in which of the following stages?"

   a. denial

   b. depression

   c. anger

   d. bargaining

17. Which of the following is *not* a goal when working with disabled persons?

   a. to help that person overcome their disability and become "normal" again

   b. to promote maximum self-care and independence within the limits of their condition

   c. to provide personal care and home maintenance services

   d. to provide relief to family members of the disabled person

18. A defense mechanism that places the blame on others or attributes one's own feelings to others is known as:

   a. repression

   b. rationalization

   c. aggression

   d. projection

19. You are caring for Lois, who has been discharged from a mental health unit. She has had a previous suicide attempt. The second week you are caring for her she states, "Nobody cares about me. I wonder if anyone would miss me when I'm not here." Your first response should be to:

   a. tell her that you would miss her and so would a lot of other people

   b. tell her she won't get better if she talks like that

   c. ask her if she is thinking about hurting herself, and report this information to your case manager

   d. report this information to her family when they arrive

20. Which of these statements describes good body mechanics?

   a. carry heavy objects as far away from the body as possible

   b. bend the knees when lifting an object off the floor

   c. bend over at the waist when lifting an object from the floor

   d. lift rather than push an object

21. The most important thing you can do to prevent the spread of disease is:

   a. wash hands before and after client contact

   b. use Lysol in the bathroom

   c. cover your mouth when coughing

   d. use sterile dressings on wounds

22. When you are working with a mentally ill person who becomes hostile, the *first* concern should be:

   a. getting the client's medications

   b. maintaining your own safety

   c. protecting the client's feelings

   d. moving the furniture

23. The recommended time to leave a glass thermometer in the mouth is:

   a. 3 minutes

   b. 1 minute

   c. 6 minutes

   d. 9 minutes

24. Mark the following lifesaving activities in the order of what should be done first. (Rank 1–4)

   ____ seek medical help

   ____ rescue the person if he or she is in danger

   ____ keep checking the person until help arrives

   ____ control bleeding

25. When assisting someone who is choking, you would first check to see if they can:

   a. move their head

   b. try to calm down

   c. place their arms around their upper abdomen

   d. cough and/or speak

26. What safety measures should you take when using cleaning products?

   a. store them only in their original containers

   b. use only well-known brands

   c. keep them in a dark place

   d. throw away the unused portion after each use

27. Clients sometimes express religious beliefs with which you might not agree. In these situations, which of these understandings should you use as a guide?

    a. you should pretend to have the same beliefs that the client has

    b. clients should be told not to discuss their beliefs with aides

    c. clients have a right to their own beliefs, which should be respected

    d. you should explain your own beliefs to the client

28. Which statement about the elderly is true?

    a. most elderly people are senile

    b. the majority of elderly live in nursing homes

    c. the elderly can learn new things

    d. the elderly have a need for dependence

29. For a rectal temperature, the thermometer should be inserted how far into the rectum?

    a. so that only the bulb tip of the thermometer is in the rectum

    b. so that the entire thermometer, except for the very end, is well inside the anus

    c. until resistance is felt

    d. about one inch

30. Why is the thumb *not* used for taking a client's pulse?

    a. the flat part of the thumb is less sensitive than the flat parts of the other fingertips

    b. the thumb can place too much pressure on the client's pulse

    c. the thumb's pulse may be felt instead of the client's pulse

    d. the thumb is more awkward to use

31. A client is receiving oxygen through a nasal tube. What safety precautions should you take?

    a. keep the television at least 5 feet away from the oxygen tank

    b. do not permit the client to drink milk

    c. do no allow candles in the client's room

    d. do not use any lotions that contain oil in the client's care

32. Mrs. Founder is in the final stages of terminal cancer. She has been unconscious for 2 days. Which of these measures should you take?

    a. do not talk to her while you are doing care

    b. turn her from side to side every 2 hours

    c. keep the draperies closed

    d. give only clear liquids to drink

33. Geneva Adams, a homemaker/home health aide, is assigned to care for Mrs. Blake. Ms. Adams notices that she feels very angry when she is with Mrs. Blake. What should Ms. Adams do?

    a. tell Mrs. Blake how she is feeling

    b. find out if other aides have experienced the same thing

    c. talk with Mrs. Blake as little as possible

    d. talk with the case manager about the situation

34. If a client needs help to do exercises, this is called:

    a. active range of motion

    b. assisted range of motion

    c. passive range of motion

    d. stable range of motion

35. Before leaving an infant alone in a crib, which action is *essential*?

    a. cover the infant

    b. put a toy in the crib

    c. raise the crib sides

    d. move all other furniture out of reach of the infant

36. In disciplining a young child, what idea is most important for you to communicate to the child?

    a. "I don't like what you have done, but I do like you."

    b. "What you have done is wrong, and you are bad."

    c. "You have to understand that you can't do everything you want to do."

    d. "You must do what you are told or you will be punished."

37. When helping Mr. Carter from the bed to the wheelchair, which of these actions is *essential*?

    a. place the foot supports of the wheelchair so his feet reach them

    b. have a plastic pad placed in the wheelchair

    c. have the brakes on the wheelchair in a locked position

    d. place a pillow on the seat for comfort

38. Mr. Carter has an indwelling catheter attached to a drainage bag. The drainage bag should always be kept:

    a. below the level of his bladder

    b. at the level of his bladder

    c. 12 inches above the bladder level

    d. attached to the bedside bars

39. If a low-salt diet is prescribed, which of these foods would be considered appropriate?

    a. olives

    b. green salad

    c. pizza

    d. slice of sandwich meat

40. Which of these fluids would be restricted for a client who is on a low-fat diet?

    a. whole milk

    b. skim milk

    c. tomato juice

    d. pineapple juice

41. Which practice is likely to help *most* to increase the food intake of a client who has a poor appetite?

    a. serving larger than average portions of preferred food at regular times

    b. serving foods that are easily digestible when the client asks for something to eat

    c. serving small amounts of nourishing foods that are liked at frequent intervals

    d. serving hot foods hot and cold foods cold

42. The best principle to follow when caring for a client with an infectious disease is to:

    a. wear a gown, gloves, and mask

    b. wait until the case manager tells you what the diagnosis is

    c. use the same infection-control measures on all people

    d. use strict isolation techniques

43. Mrs. Swenson has not had a bowel move-ment for 3 days. She has always given herself an enema if she does not have a bowel movement for that long a time. Mrs. Swenson asks you to give her an enema. What should you do?

    a. give Mrs. Swenson an enema

    b. tell Mrs. Swenson to wait another day

    c. suggest that Mrs. Swenson take a laxa-tive first

    d. contact the case manager to discuss the situation

44. When clients do not have enough fluids, which of these problems may develop?

    a. diarrhea

    b. constipation

    c. swelling

    d. gout

Mark each statement T(true) or F(false).

45. __ A person living with a chemically depen-dent person may unknowingly be assist-ing that person to remain chemically dependent.

46. __ Basic physical needs must be met before people will strive for higher psychologi-cal needs.

47. __ People with disabilities have different basic needs.

48. __ The homemaker/home health aide may change his or her assignment list, de-pending on the client's needs that day.

49. __ As one grows older, the capacity for learning decreases.

50. __ Disabled people will never be able to help themselves.

51. __ The mouth, tongue, teeth, and stomach are part of the digestive system.

52. __ Alcoholism can be a chronic and pro-gressive illness.

SECTION THREE
Quizzes

QUIZ A

Mark each statement T (true) or F (false)

1. __ If you are unsure of the correct terminology to use on the medical record, you should notify your case manager and ask for assistance.

2. __ You seem to be having a difficult time getting to know your client and are hesistant to do things for him. You should report this to your case manager.

3. __ The client insists that you give her a tub bath, even though the Plan of Care states that she should have a sponge bath. This should be reported to the agency before the change is made.

4. __ Mrs. Doe states that she doesn't feel like eating the breakfast you have prepared. Your documentation should state that client is a picky eater.

5. __ You should always document fact.

6. __ Clients may not read their medical records.

7. __ Subjective reporting means that you did not actually see something, but it was told to you.

8. __ You accidentally break a coffee cup belonging to your client. There is no need to fill out an accident report.

9. __ You see that it is getting much more difficult to transfer the client into the bathtub. This should be reported to your case manager.

10. __ While you are at your agency, you tell anyone who will listen to you how your client's daughter was in trouble with the law. This is acting in an ethical manner.

QUIZ B

Mark each statement T (true) or F (false).

1. __ A homemaker/home health aide needs orientation to the client and the plan of care.

2. __ One of the duties of a homemaker/home health aide is to give insulin to the client when the family member is unable.

3. __ Anyone of any age can give home care with little or no training as long as the individual is comfortable with the job.

4. __ One of the services a client might receive is speech therapy.

5. __ When you find a home situation unsafe, you should correct the situation without any discussion with the case manager.

6. __ If you are going to be delayed in reaching the client's home, you should notify the agency.

7. __ When a family member asks you to do something you are unable to do, you should try to complete the service as best you can.

8. __ You may give the client an aspirin from your personal supply.

9. __ Simple meal preparation may need to be done for some clients.

10. __ You should notify the case manager if the family member states that the client no longer needs home care.

11. __ You might see two or more clients in one day.

12. __ The client's personal belongings need to be treated carefully and with respect.

QUIZ C

Mark each statement T (true) or F (false).

1. __ A chronic illness is sudden and doesn't last very long.

2. __ Many individuals with disabilities will be able to tell you what you need to do for them.

3. __ It is okay to do everything for clients while you are there because it would take forever to let them do it for themselves.

4. __ Defense mechanisms, such as withdrawal and anger, are harmful to the client who uses these all the time.

5. __ Chemical dependency is a disease that can be treated.

6. __ Mentally retarded individuals cannot learn to read.

7. __ Acute illness comes on suddenly and has a short duration.

8. __ People with physical disabilities may display periods of hopelessness.

9. __ People with mental illness are not really ill.

10. __ You may not always be able to meet all the needs of the mentally ill person.

QUIZ D

Mark each statement T (true) or F (false).

1. __ It is permissible to smoke in your client's home when you need to be there for more than four hours.

2. __ A family member asks you to lend them some money because "things are tight right now." You are permitted to do this.

3. __ It is important for you as a homemaker/home health aide to present a positive attitude toward the client and the family.

4. __ You saw a visiting neighbor take something from your client's jewelry box. You need not call your case manager because this is none of your business.

5. __ You are asked by one of the family members to stay longer with the client. You should call your case manager.

QUIZ E

Fill in the blank.

1. A ———————— or ———————— is a nurse who is licensed by the state to practice.

2. An ———————— ———————— is a long-term problem.

3. A ———————— ———————— ———————— is a facility for just the elderly patient.

4. A ———————— ———————— ———————— ———————— works with the client the most.

5. ———————— are studies done to determine the numbers of days of hospitalization necessary for certain medical conditions.

QUIZ F

Fill in the blank.

1. A ———————— ———————— way of communication is to touch your client's hand gently.

2. The abbreviation tid means ———————— ———————— ————————.

3. The use of special words and abbreviations in health care is called ———————— ————————.

QUIZ G

Match the statement in Column I to the correct term in Column II.

Column I	Column II
_____ 1. expressive quality of voice that gives meaning	a. body language
_____ 2. communication without words	b. communication
_____ 3. sending and receiving of information	c. tone
_____ 4. inability to speak or use words correctly	d. pitch
_____ 5. highness or lowness of a voice	e. nonverbal expression
_____ 6. a feeling of anger	f. hostility
_____ 7. a smile, frown, or arm motion	g. apathy
_____ 8. complete lack of interest	h. aphasia
_____ 9. a syllable or word that appears at the beginning of a term	i. suffix
_____ 10. a syllable or word that appears at the end of a term	j. prefix
	k. dysphagia

QUIZ H

Circle the correct answer.

1. Who plays an important role in giving emotional support to a client?

   a. clergy

   b. family members

   c. friends

   d. members of the home care team

   e. b and c

   f. a and b

   g. d only

   h. all of the above

2. When illness strikes a family, it can cause:

   a. anxiety

   b. worry

   c. financial loss

   d. all of the above

3. When a client seems to be very apathetic about their plan of care, you should:

   a. assume they are ill

   b. forget about it

   c. notify your case manager

   d. tell a family member

4. A person who is confined to bed for long periods can develop:

   a. contractures

   b. atrophy

   c. constipation

   d. all of the above

5. Alzheimer's disease affects people:

   a. 16 to 24 years old

   b. who are mentally ill

   c. generally people between 40 and 70 years of age

   d. who are injured by a blow to the head

SECTION FOUR
Case Studies

UNIT 2

Scenario

You are scheduled to be at work at 7:30 AM to see your first client of the day. You have a total of three clients to see all day.

Your life at home has been miserable. You don't want to go to work. You are angry and preoccupied.

Questions

1. Discuss the need for employees to be at the client's home.
2. Discuss feelings of being preoccupied and what dangers or potential dangers can occur.
3. How do you think employment policies should be presented?
4. Whom can you talk to about your feelings?

UNIT 2

Scenario

You are very comfortable working with people on a one-to-one basis. Family involvement (a situation that might involve more extended family members) is a bit frightening.

Questions

1. What if someone in the family presses you for information about the client?
2. What is your responsibility?
3. What about the client?
4. What about your responsibilities?

UNIT 3

Scenario

You have held a variety of jobs and basically you did well and always left a position on a positive note. You are enrolled in a home health aide course and the instructor has presented the course objectives. Taking tests and knowing that you have to "chart" for your clients in their records and understand some of the legal involvements disturbs you. You are not sure if you really want this.

Questions

1. Do you think you should continue?
2. Who could ease your fears?
3. Review study habits.
4. Discuss self-esteem.

UNITS 3 AND 4

Scenario

You arrive at your client's home and you have a feeling that something is not quite right. You are supposed to be there for 4 hours doing personal care, light housekeeping, and laundry duties. This client needs a home health aide twice a week for 4 hours at a time. You have known this client for about one month. You have never met any member of the family. You don't *see* anything unusual, but the client tells you that "they" have decided that your services are no longer needed.

Questions

1. What do you think might have prompted your feeling?
2. What responsibility do homemaker/home health aides have to
   a. the client
   b. the agency
   c. themselves
3. Who are "they"?
4. How would you report your feeling that something is not quite right?

UNIT 5

Scenario

You are a very quiet individual and enjoy being with people. You are not a great conversationalist and you have been told this many times, but people do enjoy your company. You have never been in a position where verbal communication skills have been so emphasized as they are in home care. You also have never been in a position to deal with someone who had some physical and/or emotional barriers to communication. You are concerned.

Questions

1. What does communication mean?
2. What are barriers?
3. Can this situation be resolved? Who might be able to help you?
4. Try to name a position where communication is *not* necessary.

UNIT 5

Scenario

Mr. V. is a 51-year-old male of Laotian heritage. He has lived in this country for 15 years after leaving his homeland and spending time in refugee camps. His wife came with him, but his children did not come to America. He needs home care 2 days a week, 4 hours a day because of his multiple sclerosis. He began having symptoms 1 year ago and was forced to take a disability leave from his job as a printing press operator. At times, he would experience episodes of falling and severe upper extremity weakness. His employer was very supportive, but due to extended absence, he took permanent disability leave. He worked for this company since his arrival in the United States. His wife started a daycare center with two other women in the neighborhood. Her work takes her outside the home from 6 AM to 4 PM.

Mr. V. has lost 10 pounds in the past 2 months and has been refusing to let you or the case manager help with personal care or any cooking or housekeeping duties. Mrs. V. is becoming more frustrated and exhausted.

Questions

1. What can you do *at the time* Mr. V. refuses care?
2. What do you think the case manager could do to help
   a. Mr. V.
   b. Mrs. V.
   c. You
3. Discuss some of the cultural differences and frustrations that Mr. V. could be feeling.
4. Who else (perhaps someone from outside the home care agency) could be beneficial in helping all the people involved with this case?

UNIT 16

Scenario

Mrs. C. has been a client of your agency for a long time. She has had diabetes for many years, and has faithfully followed a proper diet, which you prepare for her 3 days a week. You prepare meals, do light housekeeping, and assist with personal care. The nurse case manager comes in and gives Mrs. C. her insulin between 7:30 and 8:00 AM Monday through Friday. Mrs. C.'s nephew, who lives three houses away, gives Mrs. C. her insulin at the other times.

Mrs. C. is having some troubling thoughts about getting worse and possibly needing more care. When you arrive one day, you find Mrs. C. crying because she was trying to cut her toenails and she couldn't see very well and now she has a deep cut on the inside of the big toe. She is very afraid that now she'll lose her leg. She's afraid to say anything to the nurse or her nephew.

Questions

1. Should you notify the case manager? Why?
2. Who should notify the nephew?
3. Are Mrs. C.'s fears unfounded? Why? Why not?
4. What might be done to treat Mrs. C.'s toe?

UNIT 18

Scenario

Mrs. L. is a 45-year-old woman who has rheumatoid arthritis in an advanced stage. She has two grown children attending college in another state. Her husband is a successful stock broker who has stated that all household chores belong to his wife. She has never been employed outside the home but has always been active in community and church functions. She has been experiencing a great deal of frustration because of her inability to continue her life as it was before.

A few weeks ago, as she was preparing for a large dinner party at her home, she fell from a stepstool and sustained fractures to her lower right leg and lower left arm. She has a full leg cast and a full arm cast. She is to be discharged from the hospital soon and will receive home care 5 days a week for 6 hours a day. She is worried about the time when her husband takes over these duties.

Questions

1. What will be the emotional impact of her fractures?
2. What physical care might be necessary for Mrs. L.?
3. Who should teach her husband to perform household tasks?
4. How could you help Mrs. L. keep in contact with her volunteer activities?

UNITS 21, 22, 23, 24

Scenario

You are really excited about being a home health aide. You have never done anything like this before. This type of work appears (from all you've learned about home care) to meet your employment needs. However, the one thing that concerns you is that you might be expected to cook and do light housekeeping. You are able to meet these needs for yourself, but this aspect of caring for a client really is bothering you.

Questions

1. Are these feelings unfounded?
2. Who can you talk to about this?
3. What can you do to help ease these feelings?
4. Whom can you go to for further information?

Scenario

Mr. F. is a 30-year-old computer sales executive in a mid-sized community. He was involved in an automobile accident one month ago. He is single and lives in a modest one-story home. The accident resulted in paralysis of his legs. His family has been supportive, but as discharge from the hospital approaches, Mr. F. is frightened about returning home.

Home care is arranged by social services for Mr. F. and you are assigned to Mr. F. 7 days a week, 4 hours a day to help with personal care, meal management, cleaning duties, and assistance in rehabilitation care. Family members have arranged to be there for Mr. F. when you cannot be.

Questions

1. Describe the fears Mr. F. might have about returning home.

2. What personal care might be needed for Mr. F.?

3. What other members of the home care team could possibly be involved with Mr. F.?

4. What could family members provide for Mr. F.?

5. What types of education does Mr. F. need?

SECTION FIVE
Competency Checklists

In some cases, disposable gloves must be used when certain procedures are done (usually any procedure in which the caregiver comes in contact with any body fluids). The home health aide should always ask an agency representative (case manager or nurse) when and how often these supplies will be provided.

Not all clients will have adjustable or hospital beds. Allowances will have to be made for some procedures. (If a hospital hi-low bed is used, the wheels and brakes need to be locked when moving the client.) Siderails need to be in the correct position.

For all procedures, the client should be given privacy. Every household has different areas where a client spends the majority of his or her time. For example, some client areas are in the living room because it might be the largest area where family members can help give care and yet enjoy TV, stereo, and so on with the client.

Many times a family member is a designated caregiver for certain specialized procedures that are beyond the limitations of a homemaker/home health aide. Always check with the case manager and the plan of care.

PROCEDURE 1: TESTING BLOOD

All items must be successfully completed in this skill. The practice column is for student/partner use. The instructor will check, date, and initial the other two columns.

Practice	*Satisfactory*	*Unsatisfactory*	*Procedural Steps*
_____	_____	_____	1. Gather necessary equipment: glucose meter apparatus blood lancet (sharp prick) gloves alcohol swab and cotton ball watch with second hand blood strips—be sure that you have blood strips that correspond with your glucometer. Also check to see that the blood strips are not outdated.
_____	_____	_____	2. Cleanse the side of a distal finger with alcohol, then squeeze the finger and prick the finger with the lancet. Wipe away the first drop of blood. You may also use a special apparatus to prick the finger. Rotate fingers if doing this procedure daily.
_____	_____	_____	3. With palm facing down, firmly apply pressure to the pricked finger until a large drop of hanging blood forms. Bring the blood strip to the finger and touch the blood strip to the drop of blood. Completely cover the test zone of the strip with the blood. Wear gloves when doing the testing for infection control purposes.
_____	_____	_____	4. Insert blood strip into machine and observe read-out.
_____	_____	_____	5. Record reading and discard blood strip in proper container.

PROCEDURE 2: HANDWASHING

All items must be successfully completed in this skill. The practice column is for student/partner use. The instructor will check, date, and initial the other two columns.

Practice	Satisfactory	Unsatisfactory	Procedural Steps
_____	_____	_____	1. Collect the items needed for handwashing and bring them to the bathroom or kitchen sink: soap soap dish towel (paper towels preferred) washbasin (if needed) orange stick (optional)
_____	_____	_____	2. Using a clean paper towel turn on water and adjust temperature. Wet hands with fingertips pointing down.
_____	_____	_____	3. Apply soap—either liquid or bar.
_____	_____	_____	4. With fingertips pointing down, lather well. Rub your hands together in a circular motion to generate friction. Wash carefully between your fingers and rub fingernails against the palm of the other hand to force soap under the nails. Keep washing for 10 to 15 seconds. Be sure to clean under fingernails.
_____	_____	_____	5. With fingertips still pointing down, rinse all the soap off. Be careful not to lean against the side of the sink or touch the inside of the sink because germs are there.
_____	_____	_____	6. With clean paper towel or cloth hand towel, dry hands. Take clean paper towel and turn off faucet. Do not turn off faucet with clean hands because the faucet handles are contaminated.
_____	_____	_____	7. Discard the paper towel in the wastebasket. Hand towels can be placed in a laundry hamper.
_____	_____	_____	8. Apply hand lotion if hands are dry or chapped.

PROCEDURE 3: GLOVING

All items must be successfully completed in this skill. The practice column is for student/partner use. The instructor will check, date, and initial the other two columns.

Practice	Satisfactory	Unsatisfactory	Procedural Steps
_____	_____	_____	1. Wash your hands.
_____	_____	_____	2. With your dominant hand, usually the right, pull out one glove and slide it on to your other hand.
_____	_____	_____	3. With the gloved hand, pull out another glove and slide your dominant hand into it.
_____	_____	_____	4. Interlace your fingers to make the gloves comfortable and adjust the top of the gloves to stay flat.

Removal of Contaminated Gloves

Practice	Satisfactory	Unsatisfactory	
_____	_____	_____	1. Use your dominant hand to grasp the opposite glove on the palm side, about 1 inch below the wrist.
_____	_____	_____	2. Pull the glove down and off so that it is removed inside out and keep hold of that glove with the fingertips of the gloved hands.
_____	_____	_____	3. Using your ungloved hand, insert the fingers into the inside of the remaining glove down and off, inside out, so that the glove you are holding with your fingertips is now inside the glove that you are taking off.
_____	_____	_____	4. Drop both soiled gloves together into waste receptacle (which is a double bag).
_____	_____	_____	5. Wash your hands.

PROCEDURE 4: PUTTING ON AND REMOVING PERSONAL PROTECTIVE EQUIPMENT

All items must be successfully completed in this skill. The practice column is for student/partner use. The instructor will check, date, and initial the other two columns.

Practice	*Satisfactory*	*Unsatisfactory*	*Procedural Steps*
_____	_____	_____	1. Assemble personal protective equipment.
_____	_____	_____	2. Remove wristwatch and place on clean paper towel.
_____	_____	_____	3. Wash your hands.
_____	_____	_____	4. First piece of equipment to apply will be the mask.
_____	_____	_____	5. Adjust the mask over your nose and mouth. Tie the top strings first and then the bottom strings. Your mask must always be dry, so that droplets are not absorbed into the paper of the mask. If the mask becomes wet, you must replace it.
_____	_____	_____	6. Unfold and open the gown, so that you can slide your arms into the sleeves and your hands come right through. Slip the fingers of both hands inside the neckband of the gown and grasp the two strings at the back and tie into a bow, so that they can be undone easily after the procedure is completed. Reach behind you, overlap the two edges of the gown so that your uniform is completely covered and then secure the waist ties.
_____	_____	_____	7. **Remember:** Your moisture-resistant gown is only worn once and is then discarded in a container for contaminated linen.

Removing Contaminated Gown and Mask

_____	_____	_____	1. Undo the waist ties of your gown.
_____	_____	_____	2. Wash hands.
_____	_____	_____	3. Undo your mask, bottom ties first, then top ties. Holding top ties, drop mask in appropriate waste receptacle.

Practice	Satisfactory	Unsatisfactory	Procedural Steps
_____	_____	_____	4. Undo neckties and loosen gown at shoulder.
_____	_____	_____	5. Slip finger of right hand inside left cuff without touching outside of gown and pull gown over left hand. With your gown-covered left hand, pull gown down over right hand and then right arm.
_____	_____	_____	6. Fold gown with contaminated side inward and dispose of it into the appropriate receptacle.
_____	_____	_____	7. Wash hands.
_____	_____	_____	8. Remove watch from paper towel and place back on wrist.

All items must be successfully completed in this skill. The practice column is for student/partner use. The instructor will check, date, and initial the other two columns.

Practice	Satisfactory	Unsatisfactory	Procedural Steps
_____	_____	_____	1. Assemble equipment: clean specimen container, cover, label paper towels gloves plastic transport bag
_____	_____	_____	2. Fill in label with client's name, date, time, and type of specimen.
_____	_____	_____	3. Remove cover from the container and place all the equipment on the clean paper towel.
_____	_____	_____	4. Wash your hands and put on gloves.
_____	_____	_____	5. With gloved hands, pick up the specimen and place it in the container so that you do not contaminate any part of the container.
_____	_____	_____	6. Remove gloves and wash hands.
_____	_____	_____	7. Using the paper towel, pick up the container without touching it with your bare hands.
_____	_____	_____	8. Place the container in the plastic bag and seal it.
_____	_____	_____	9. Send specimen to the laboratory per instruction of your nurse supervisor.

PROCEDURE 6: MAINTAINING BODY ALIGNMENT

All items must be successfully completed in this skill. The practice column is for student/partner use. The instructor will check, date, and initial the other two columns.

Practice	*Satisfactory*	*Unsatisfactory*	*Procedural Steps*
_____	_____	_____	1. Observe alignment of client in sitting or lying position.
_____	_____	_____	2. If sitting up—is head erect and spine in straight alignment?
_____	_____	_____	3. If sitting up—is body weight evenly distributed on buttocks and thighs?
_____	_____	_____	4. If sitting up—are feet supported on floor and are ankles comfortably flexed?
_____	_____	_____	5. If sitting up—are forearms supported on armrest, or on lap, or on table in front of chair?
_____	_____	_____	6. If lying on side—are pillows and positioning supports correctly placed?
_____	_____	_____	7. If lying on side—is spinal column in correct alignment?
_____	_____	_____	8. If lying on side—are arms positioned over the chest?

All items must be successfully completed in this skill. The practice column is for student/partner use. The instructor will check, date, and initial the other two columns.

Practice	Satisfactory	Unsatisfactory	Procedural Steps
_____	_____	_____	1. Wash your hands.
_____	_____	_____	2. Tell client what you are going to do.
_____	_____	_____	3. Lift client's far leg and cross it over the leg that is nearest you.
_____	_____	_____	4. Lift the far arm over the chest, bend the elbow, and bring the hand toward the client's shoulder.
_____	_____	_____	5. Place the hand nearest the head of the bed on the far shoulder and place your other hand on the client's hip on the far side.
_____	_____	_____	6. Brace your thighs against the side of the bed and smoothly roll client toward you. Make sure that the client's upper leg comes over and bend it at the knee to ensure that the new position is stable.
_____	_____	_____	7. Go to opposite side of bed and place your hands over the client's shoulder and pull upper body to the center of the bed. Place your hands over client's hips and pull the rest of the client's body to the center of the bed and into good body alignment.
_____	_____	_____	8. Place a pillow against the client's back and secure it by pushing part under the client's back.
_____	_____	_____	9. Support the knee, ankle, and foot of the upper leg with a pillow, which also prevents the knees and ankles from rubbing against each other and causing skin irritation. Cover client.
_____	_____	_____	10. Wash your hands.
_____	_____	_____	11. Document procedure completion, time, and client's reaction.

PROCEDURE 8: MOVING THE CLIENT UP IN BED USING THE DRAWSHEET

All items must be successfully completed in this skill. The practice column is for student/partner use. The instructor will check, date, and initial the other two columns.

Practice	*Satisfactory*	*Unsatisfactory*	*Procedural Steps*
_____	_____	_____	1. Wash your hands.
_____	_____	_____	2. Tell client what you plan to do. Have your partner stand on the opposite side of the bed to assist you.
_____	_____	_____	3. Place pillow at the head of the bed to protect the client's head. Roll both sides of the drawsheet or flat sheet folded in fours toward the client. Place the client's feet 12 inches apart, so that they will not bump together as you move the client.
_____	_____	_____	4. With the hand nearest the client's feet, firmly grasp the rolled drawsheet or folded sheet. With the other hand, both of you cradle the client's head and shoulders and firmly grasp the top of the rolled drawsheet or folded sheet.
_____	_____	_____	5. Turn your body and feet toward the head of the bed. Keep your feet about 12 inches apart and bend your knees slightly to achieve good body mechanics as you lift the client.
_____	_____	_____	6. Coordinate your lift—on the count of three, together lift the drawsheet and the client toward the head of the bed without dragging the client. Align the client's body and limbs so that the client is straight and comfortable.
_____	_____	_____	7. Place the pillow back under the client's head and tighten the drawsheet. Replace the covers and make the client comfortable.
_____	_____	_____	8. Wash your hands.
_____	_____	_____	9. Document completion of the procedure, time, and client's reaction.

PROCEDURE 9:   LOG ROLLING THE CLIENT

All items must be successfully completed in this skill. The practice column is for student/partner use. The instructor will check, date, and initial the other two columns.

Practice	Satisfactory	Unsatisfactory		Procedural Steps
_____	_____	_____	1.	Wash your hands.
_____	_____	_____	2.	Tell client what you plan to do.
_____	_____	_____	3.	With both you and your helper on the same side of the bed, remove the top covers.
_____	_____	_____	4.	Place your hand and arm under the client's head and shoulder. Your helper places his arms under the client's body and legs. On the count of three, lift the client toward you as a single unit.
_____	_____	_____	5.	Do not allow the client to bend and use good body mechanics yourselves by bending your knees and keeping your backs straight.
_____	_____	_____	6.	Place a pillow lengthwise between the client's thighs and legs and fold the client's arms over the chest.
_____	_____	_____	7.	Go over to the other side of the bed. You are in a position to keep the shoulders and upper body straight and your helper is positioned to keep the client's lower body, hips, and legs straight. Reach over the client and roll the drawsheet firmly against the client. On the count of three, the client is rolled toward you in a single movement, keeping the client's head, spine, and legs in a straight position.
_____	_____	_____	8.	To maintain the client's new position and alignment, place pillows against the spine and leave the pillow between the client's legs. Other small pillows or folded towels can be placed under the client's head and neck and under the arms for support.
_____	_____	_____	9.	Fold the drawsheet back over the pillows supporting the spine. Make sure the client's alignment is straight and that the client is comfortable. Arrange covers for the client.
_____	_____	_____	10.	Wash your hands.
_____	_____	_____	11.	Record this repositioning, time, and any observation you made.

All items must be successfully completed in this skill. The practice column is for student/partner use. The instructor will check, date, and initial the other two columns.

Practice	Satisfactory	Unsatisfactory	Procedural Steps
_____	_____	_____	1. Wash your hands.
_____	_____	_____	2. Tell client what you plan to do.
_____	_____	_____	3. Place pillow under the client's head, so that the client's head is about 2 inches above the level of the bed. The pillow should extend slightly under the shoulders.
_____	_____	_____	4. Have client's arms extended straight out with palms of the hands flat on the bed. The arms can be supported by pillows or covered foam pads placed under the forearms and extending from just above the elbows to the ends of the fingers.
_____	_____	_____	5. Place a small pillow or rolled towel along the side of the client's thighs and tuck part of the support under the thigh, ensuring that the part under the thighs is smooth. This maintains alignment of the hips and thighs and helps prevent the hips from rotating outward or externally.
_____	_____	_____	6. Place a pillow under the back of the ankle to relieve pressure on the heels.
_____	_____	_____	7. Wash your hands.
_____	_____	_____	8. Document the time and position change and the client's reaction.

PROCEDURE 11: POSITIONING THE CLIENT IN LATERAL/SIDE-LYING POSITION

All items must be successfully completed in this skill. The practice column is for student/partner use. The instructor will check, date, and initial the other two columns.

Practice	*Satisfactory*	*Unsatisfactory*	*Procedural Steps*
_____	_____	_____	1. Wash your hands.
_____	_____	_____	2. Tell client what you plan to do.
_____	_____	_____	3. Go to opposite side of bed from the direction you are planning to turn the client toward.
_____	_____	_____	4. Cross the client's arms over the chest. Place your arm under the client's neck and shoulders. Place your other arm under the client's midback. Move the upper part of the client's body toward you.
_____	_____	_____	5. Place one arm under the client's waist and the other under the thighs. Move the lower part of the client's body toward you.
_____	_____	_____	6. Turn client to opposite side. Pull shoulder that is touching the bed slightly toward you. Pull buttock that is touching the bed slightly toward you. Place pillow under back and buttocks. Place bottom leg in extension and flex upper leg. Place small folded blanket or pillow between the upper and lower leg.
_____	_____	_____	7. Place pillow under client's head. Rotate the upper arm to bring it up to the pillow with the palm facing up. Place the other arm on a pillow that extends from above the elbow to the fingers. Extend the fingers.
_____	_____	_____	8. Check the client's position to see if the body is in good vertical alignment.
_____	_____	_____	9. Wash your hands.
_____	_____	_____	10. Document time, change of position, and client's reaction.

PROCEDURE 12: POSITIONING THE CLIENT IN PRONE POSITION

All items must be successfully completed in this skill. The practice column is for student/partner use. The instructor will check, date, and initial the other two columns.

Practice	Satisfactory	Unsatisfactory	Procedural Steps
_____	_____	_____	1. Wash your hands.
_____	_____	_____	2. Tell client what you plan to do.
_____	_____	_____	3. Turn client on abdomen. Check to see if spine is straight and face is turned to either side.
_____	_____	_____	4. Legs are extended. Arms are flexed and brought up to either side of head.
_____	_____	_____	5. A small pillow can be placed under the abdomen, especially for women as this reduces pressure against their breasts. An alternative method is to roll a small towel and place it under shoulders to reduce pressure.
_____	_____	_____	6. Place another pillow under lower legs to prevent pressure on toes.
_____	_____	_____	7. Client can also be moved to foot of bed so feet extend over mattress. This is an alternative method for preventing pressure on toes.
_____	_____	_____	8. Wash your hands.
_____	_____	_____	9. Document time, position change, and client's reaction.

PROCEDURE 13: POSITIONING THE CLIENT IN FOWLER'S POSITION

All items must be successfully completed in this skill. The practice column is for student/partner use. The instructor will check, date, and initial the other two columns.

Practice	Satisfactory	Unsatisfactory	Procedural Steps
_____	_____	_____	1. Wash your hands.
_____	_____	_____	2. Tell the client what you plan to do.
_____	_____	_____	3. Check to see if the client's spine and legs are straight and in the middle of the bed.
_____	_____	_____	4. Support client's head and neck with one, two, or three pillows. If client has a hospital bed, raise bed to 45° angle.
_____	_____	_____	5. Knees may be flexed and supported with small pillows.
_____	_____	_____	6. Pillows may be placed under each arm from elbows to fingertips to support shoulders.
_____	_____	_____	7. Place pillow or padded footboard against feet.
_____	_____	_____	8. Wash your hands.
_____	_____	_____	9. Document time, position change, and client's reaction.

PROCEDURE 14: ASSISTING THE CLIENT FROM BED TO CHAIR

All items must be successfully completed in this skill. The practice column is for student/partner use. The instructor will check, date, and initial the other two columns.

Practice	Satisfactory	Unsatisfactory		Procedural Steps
_____	_____	_____	1.	Wash your hands.
_____	_____	_____	2.	Tell the client what you plan to do.
_____	_____	_____	3.	Assemble needed equipment: wheelchair transfer belt client's shoes and socks
_____	_____	_____	4.	Place chair so client moves toward client's strongest side. Set chair at 45°angle to bed. Lock wheels.
_____	_____	_____	5.	Assist client to sit at edge of bed.
_____	_____	_____	6.	Wait a few seconds to allow the client to adjust to sitting position. Assist client to put on shoes and socks.
_____	_____	_____	7.	Apply transfer belt. Make sure the belt is not too tight or too loose.
_____	_____	_____	8.	Spread your feet apart and flex your hips and knees, aligning your knees with client's.
_____	_____	_____	9.	Grasp transfer belt from underneath. Rock the client up to standing on the count of three while straightening your hips and legs, keeping knees slightly flexed.
_____	_____	_____	10.	If client has a weak leg, press your knee against it or block client's foot with yours to prevent weaker leg from sliding out from under the client.
_____	_____	_____	11.	Instruct client to use armrest on chair for support and be sure to flex your hips and knees while lowering client into chair. Remove transfer belt.
_____	_____	_____	12.	Check alignment of client in chair and make adjustments accordingly.
_____	_____	_____	13.	Wash your hands.
_____	_____	_____	14.	Document time, position change, and client's reactions.

PROCEDURE 15: ASSISTING THE CLIENT FROM CHAIR TO BED

All items must be successfully completed in this skill. The practice column is for student/partner use. The instructor will check, date, and initial the other two columns.

Practice	Satisfactory	Unsatisfactory	Procedural Steps
_____	_____	_____	1. Wash your hands.
_____	_____	_____	2. Tell client what you plan to do.
_____	_____	_____	3. Position client with strong side toward bed with wheelchair at 45°angle.
_____	_____	_____	4. Apply transfer belt and place both hands on front of the belt. Instruct client, if able, to put feet flat on the floor and hands on the chair. On the count of three, have client push up to standing position. While standing, have the client pivot (turn) on strong leg toward the bed. Have the client lower himself/herself to the bed to a sitting position.
_____	_____	_____	5. Remove shoes, socks, and transfer belt. Assist the client to lying position. Position client in comfortable position and in good alignment.
_____	_____	_____	6. Wash hands.
_____	_____	_____	7. Document time, change of position, and client's reaction.

PROCEDURE 16: TRANSFERRING THE CLIENT FROM WHEELCHAIR TO TOILET/COMMODE

All items must be successfully completed in this skill. The practice column is for student/partner use. The instructor will check, date, and initial the other two columns.

Practice	Satisfactory	Unsatisfactory		Procedural Steps
_____	_____	_____	1.	Wash hands.
_____	_____	_____	2.	Tell client what you plan to do.
_____	_____	_____	3.	Have client in wheelchair with strong side nearer to the toilet or commode.
_____	_____	_____	4.	Lock the wheelchair. Apply transfer belt. Lift foot pieces out of way.
_____	_____	_____	5.	Loosen clothing on the client, but not too loose that the slacks fall while transferring.
_____	_____	_____	6.	Have client lean forward in chair and place feet apart. Have client place hands on arm-piece and on the count of three push up. Place your hand on the transfer belt.
_____	_____	_____	7.	Stand client up and have client place strong arm on grab bars. You continue to hold onto the transfer belt and slowly lower client onto the toilet or commode. Have client hang onto grab bar while you drop the client's pants.
_____	_____	_____	8.	Remove belt and move wheelchair out of way.
_____	_____	_____	9.	Provide privacy for client. Check often to see if client is all right. Give client toilet paper.
_____	_____	_____	10.	Assist the client as needed, return to wheelchair and prior activity.
_____	_____	_____	11.	Wash client's hands and your hands.
_____	_____	_____	12.	Document bowel movement or urination.

PROCEDURE 17: PERFORMING PASSIVE RANGE OF MOTION EXERCISES

All items must be successfully completed in this skill. The practice column is for student/partner use. The instructor will check, date, and initial the other two columns.

Practice	*Satisfactory*	*Unsatisfactory*	*Procedural Steps*
_____	_____	_____	1. Wash your hands.
_____	_____	_____	2. Read any special instructions for these exercises for your client.
_____	_____	_____	3. Tell client what you plan to do. Ask client to assist as much as possible.
_____	_____	_____	4. Exercise the shoulder. Supporting the upper and lower arms, exercise the shoulder joint. Abduct (away from the body) the entire arm out at right angles to the body, and then adduct (bring back to the midline of the body) the arm back to the center of the client's body.
_____	_____	_____	5. Exercise the elbow. Bend elbow, keeping the arm close to the body. Bring the fingers to touch the shoulder. Lower the fingers to touch the bed.
_____	_____	_____	6. Exercise the forearm. Bring the arm out to the side. Rest it on the bed. Take the client's hand and rotate the arm, palm up and palm down.
_____	_____	_____	7. Exercise the wrist and fingers. Take the client's hand and move the hand forward and back. Move the hand side to side. Curl the client's fingers and straighten them. Spread the fingers apart and rotate the thumb. Touch all fingers to thumb.
_____	_____	_____	8. Exercise the knee and hip while the client is lying on the back. Bend the knee and raise it to the chest. Bring the leg out to the side and back. Cross one leg over the other leg. Allow the leg to rest on the bed with the knee straight and the heel resting on the bed. Rotate the leg inward and outward.

Practice	Satisfactory	Unsatisfactory		Procedural Steps
_____	_____	_____	9.	Exercise the ankle. Bend client's knee slightly and support lower leg with one hand. With other hand, bend client's foot downward (plantar flexion) and then bend client's foot toward client's body (dorsiflexion). With client's legs extended on bed, place both hands on client's foot and move foot inward and then outward.
_____	_____	_____	10.	Exercise the toes. Bend (flexion) and straighten (extension) each toe. Do abduction and adduction with each toe as you did with the fingers.
_____	_____	_____	11.	Go to other side and repeat movements for each joint.
_____	_____	_____	12.	Wash hands.
_____	_____	_____	13.	Document the completion of the exercises and client's reactions.

All items must be successfully completed in this skill. The practice column is for student/partner use. The instructor will check, date, and initial the other two columns.

Practice	Satisfactory	Unsatisfactory	Procedural Steps
_____	_____	_____	1. Wash your hands. Apply transfer belt unless instructed not to.
_____	_____	_____	2. Always walk on the client's weak side.
_____	_____	_____	3. Walk slightly behind the client holding onto the transfer belt from behind.
_____	_____	_____	4. For the client using crutches, hold onto the transfer belt if the client feels uncomfortable using the crutches.
_____	_____	_____	5. For the client using a walker, instruct the client to place the walker firmly before walking. If the client is strong enough, the walker and the weaker leg can be moved forward at the same time.
_____	_____	_____	6. For the client using a cane, instruct the client to hold the cane in the hand opposite the weaker leg. If the right ankle has been injured, the client should hold the cane in the left hand.
_____	_____	_____	7. Balance is a judgmental situation. If the client has poor balance, the aide should support the weak side. If the client has good balance and can walk without assistive devices, the aide should use a transfer belt for safety reasons.
_____	_____	_____	8. Wash your hands at completion of the procedure.
_____	_____	_____	9. Document how far the client walked and client's reaction.

PROCEDURE 19: LIFTING THE CLIENT USING A MECHANICAL LIFT

All items must be successfully completed in this skill. The practice column is for student/partner use. The instructor will check, date, and initial the other two columns.

Practice	Satisfactory	Unsatisfactory	Procedural Steps
_____	_____	_____	1. Wash your hands and assemble equipment.
_____	_____	_____	2. Tell client what you plan to do.
_____	_____	_____	3. Position chair near bed and allow adequate room to maneuver the lift.
_____	_____	_____	4. Roll client away from you.
_____	_____	_____	5. Place hammock sling or canvas strips under client to form seat; with two canvas pieces, lower edge fits under client's knees (wide piece); upper edge goes under client's shoulders (narrow piece).
_____	_____	_____	6. Go to opposite side of bed and pull hammock or strips through.
_____	_____	_____	7. Roll client supine into canvas seat.
_____	_____	_____	8. Place lift's horseshoe bar under side of bed (on side with chair). Have base of lift in maximum open position and lock.
_____	_____	_____	9. Lower horizontal bar to sling level by releasing hydraulic valve. Lock valve.
_____	_____	_____	10. Attach hooks on strap (chain) to holes in sling. Short chains/straps hook to top holes of sling; longer chains to bottom of sling. Point hooks to the outside when attaching.
_____	_____	_____	11. Fold client's arm over the chest.
_____	_____	_____	12. Pump handle until client is raised free of bed, but no higher than necessary.
_____	_____	_____	13. Using steering handle to pull lift from bed and maneuver to chair.
_____	_____	_____	14. Roll base around chair. Slowly release check valve and lower client into chair.
_____	_____	_____	15. Check to see if client is positioned correctly. Unhook chains or straps and remove lift.

Practice	Satisfactory	Unsatisfactory		Procedural Steps
_____	_____	_____	16.	If straps are used, they can be removed. If the hammock sling is used, sling will remain underneath client so it is in position for transfer back to bed.
_____	_____	_____	17.	Wash your hands.
_____	_____	_____	18.	Document transfer, time completed, and client's reactions.

PROCEDURE 20:   ASSISTING WITH TUB BATH OR SHOWER

All items must be successfully completed in this skill. The practice column is for student/partner use. The instructor will check, date, and initial the other two columns.

Practice	Satisfactory	Unsatisfactory		Procedural Steps
_____	_____	_____	1.	If possible, plan the tub bath or shower for a time convenient for the client. A tub bath or shower should not take more than 15 minutes unless there is a special reason for a longer bath.
_____	_____	_____	2.	Assemble needed supplies and place in bathroom:
				clean clothing
				bath seat or stool
				2 washcloths and towels
				shampoo (if needed)
				plastic pitcher (if shampooing client's hair)
				hose attachment
				comb and brush
				skidproof bath mat
				soap
_____	_____	_____	3.	Wash hands.
_____	_____	_____	4.	Tell client what you plan to do.
_____	_____	_____	5.	Fill tub one-third full with warm water. **Caution:** Test the temperature with a thermometer or on inside of wrist to be sure it will not burn the client. Place a skidproof mat in the bottom of the tub. If client is taking a shower, regulate the flow and be sure the temperature is correct. The water should be about 115° F (46°C).
_____	_____	_____	6.	Assist the client to sit on a chair or on the closed toilet seat. Help the client undress. Place soiled clothing in the hamper. Close the bathroom door so the client will not be chilled.

Practice	Satisfactory	Unsatisfactory		Procedural Steps
_____	_____	_____	7.	For a tub bath, help client to sit on the edge of the tub. If there is a safety bar, have client hold onto it. When client has gained balance, help the client to turn and lift both legs into the tub. Give assistance by supporting the client under the arms and helping the client to slowly sit down in the tub facing the faucets. If the client cannot sit in the tub, place a bath stool in the water. Help the client to sit on the stool.
_____	_____	_____	8.	If the client needs a shampoo, wet the hair and rub in shampoo, lather, and massage head. If possible, have the client tilt head back. Pour water over the head using the pitcher or attach the hose to the faucet and use it to rinse the head. Repeat shampoo, massage, and rinse. Client may hold a washcloth over the eyes during the shampoo to prevent soap entering the eyes.
_____	_____	_____	9.	Give the client a washcloth and soap. Allow the client to do as much as possible. Assist as necessary. If shower is running, make sure the flow is not too heavy; check water temperature often.
_____	_____	_____	10.	Remain beside the tub at all times during the bath or shower. **Caution:** Be ready to help the client at any moment. If the client should feel faint, empty water from the tub, cover the client with a towel to avoid unnecessary chilling, and lower the client's head between the client's knees.
_____	_____	_____	11.	For a tub bath, help the client raise out of the water. Assist the client out of the water. Assist the client to sit on the edge of the tub. Bring client's legs over to outside and assist the client to stand. Allow the client to sit on the closed toilet seat or the chair.
_____	_____	_____	12.	Make certain that the client's body is thoroughly dry. Help dry difficult areas such as the back and shoulders. Be sure underarms and area under breasts are completely dry. Pay special attention to the feet. Dry soles of feet and between toes. Apply lotion to the client's skin as required.

Practice	Satisfactory	Unsatisfactory		Procedural Steps
_____	_____	_____	13.	For a shower, make sure the client is completely washed and rinsed and then turn off the shower. Towel dry and assist client out of the shower area.
_____	_____	_____	14.	Assist client to dress in clean clothes.
_____	_____	_____	15.	Help client back to bed, to a wheelchair, or to a lounge chair.
_____	_____	_____	16.	Return to the bathroom and drain and clean tub. Place dirty clothes and towels in the hamper. Put supplies away.
_____	_____	_____	17.	Wash hands.
_____	_____	_____	18.	Document procedure, any observations, and client's reaction.

All items must be successfully completed in this skill. The practice column is for student/partner use. The instructor will check, date, and initial the other two columns.

Practice	Satisfactory	Unsatisfactory		Procedural Steps
_____	_____	_____	1.	Gather supplies for the complete series of procedures including: soap and gloves washcloths and towels fresh clothes body lotion change of bed linens bath basin, two-thirds filled with water adult brief if needed
_____	_____	_____	2.	Close windows to prevent a draft from blowing on the client. Place a "Do Not Disturb" sign on the door to avoid interruptions.
_____	_____	_____	3.	Wash your hands.
_____	_____	_____	4.	Tell client what you plan to do.
_____	_____	_____	5.	Remove blankets, leaving the top sheet covering the client. Place one pillow under client's head.
_____	_____	_____	6.	Pull out bottom part of top sheet so it covers client loosely. Remove client's clothing.
_____	_____	_____	7.	Place a basin of water on the chair or dresser at the bedside.
_____	_____	_____	8.	Assist client in moving to side of bed nearest you.
_____	_____	_____	9.	Moisten washcloth, squeeze out excess water. Form a mitt by folding a washcloth around one hand.
_____	_____	_____	10.	Wash the client's eyes first. Wipe from the inner corner to the outer corner of the eye. Keep soap out of eyes. Wash the face, ears, and neck. Pat dry with the face towel.
_____	_____	_____	11.	Lift client's farthest arm and lay a bath towel under the area to keep bed dry. Wash with soap, rinse, and pat dry, making sure the arm, underarm, and hand are cleaned and thoroughly dry. Repeat for other arm. Apply underarm deodorant or bath powder if client desires.

Practice	Satisfactory	Unsatisfactory	Procedural Steps
_____	_____	_____	12. Give nail care as ordered. Trim nails *if allowed.*
_____	_____	_____	13. Place towel over client's chest, then pull sheet down to waist. Working under the towel, wash with soap, rinse, and dry chest. Rinse, dry, and powder area under a woman's breasts carefully to prevent skin irritation and redness. Replace sheet over chest.
_____	_____	_____	14. Have client bend one knee. Fold sheet up from the foot of the bed. Expose the thigh, leg, and foot. Place a towel under the area, and put the basin on the towel, placing client's foot in basin. Wash and rinse foot. Remove the foot from the basin and dry it well.
_____	_____	_____	15. Remove the basin from the bed. Follow the same procedure for the other leg and foot.
_____	_____	_____	16. Lightly apply lotion on legs and feet if skin is dry (never massage legs).
_____	_____	_____	17. Change the water in the basin before proceeding with the bath. If at any time during the bath, the water becomes dirty or cool, change it.
_____	_____	_____	18. Assist the client to move toward your side of the bed. Place bath towel lengthwise by the client's back and buttocks. Starting at the hairline use long, firm strokes while washing the back.
_____	_____	_____	19. Give the client a back rub starting at the base of the spine.
_____	_____	_____	20. Prepare washcloth with soap and have client wash the genital area, if able. Rinse the cloth and have client wipe and dry the genitals, if capable.
_____	_____	_____	21. Spread the towel under client's head and comb or brush hair.
_____	_____	_____	22. Assist the client into clean clothes.
_____	_____	_____	23. Remove the basin, dirty linens, and the other equipment away from the bed.
_____	_____	_____	24. Change the bed linens using the procedure for making an occupied bed.

Practice	Satisfactory	Unsatisfactory		Procedural Steps
_____	_____	_____	25.	Leave the client in a comfortable position. After all the activities, the client may require a rest period.
_____	_____	_____	26.	Wash your hands.
_____	_____	_____	27.	Document procedure and time, observations, and client's reaction.

PROCEDURE 22: GIVING A PARTIAL BATH

All items must be successfully completed in this skill. The practice column is for student/partner use. The instructor will check, date, and initial the other two columns.

Practice	*Satisfactory*	*Unsatisfactory*	*Procedural Steps*
_____	_____	_____	1. Gather supplies for the complete series of procedures including: soap and gloves washcloths and towels fresh clothes body lotion change of bed linens bath basin, two-thirds filled with water adult brief if needed
_____	_____	_____	2. Close windows to prevent a draft from blowing on the client. Place a "Do Not Disturb" sign on the door to avoid interruptions.
_____	_____	_____	3. Wash your hands.
_____	_____	_____	4. Tell client what you plan to do.
_____	_____	_____	5. Remove blankets, leaving the top sheet covering the client. Place one pillow under client's head.
_____	_____	_____	6. Pull out bottom part of top sheet so it covers client loosely. Remove client's clothing.
_____	_____	_____	7. Place a basin of water on the chair or dresser at the bedside.
_____	_____	_____	8. Assist client in moving to side of bed nearest you.
_____	_____	_____	9. Moisten washcloth, squeeze out excess water. Form a mitt by folding a washcloth around one hand.
_____	_____	_____	10. Wash the client's eyes first. Wipe from the inner corner to the outer corner of the eye. Keep soap out of eyes. Wash the face, ears, and neck. Pat dry with the face towel.
_____	_____	_____	11. Lift client's farthest arm and lay a bath towel under the area to keep bed dry. Wash with soap, rinse, and pat dry, making sure the arm, underarm, and hand are cleaned and thoroughly dry. Repeat for other arm. Apply underarm deodorant or bath powder if client desires.

Practice	Satisfactory	Unsatisfactory		Procedural Steps
_____	_____	_____	12.	Give nail care as ordered. Trim nails *if allowed.*
_____	_____	_____	13.	Place towel over client's chest, then pull sheet down to waist. Working under the towel, wash with soap, rinse, and dry chest. Rinse, dry, and powder area under a woman's breasts carefully to prevent skin irritation and redness. Replace sheet over chest.
_____	_____	_____	14.	Change the water in the basin before proceeding with the bath. If at any time during the bath, the water becomes dirty or cool, change it.
_____	_____	_____	15.	Assist the client to move toward your side of the bed. Place bath towel lengthwise by the client's back and buttocks. Starting at the hairline use long, firm strokes while washing the back.
_____	_____	_____	16.	Give the client a back rub starting at the base of the spine.
_____	_____	_____	17.	Prepare washcloth with soap and have client wash the genital area, if able. Rinse the cloth and have client wipe and dry the genitals, if capable.
_____	_____	_____	18.	Spread the towel under client's head and comb or brush hair.
_____	_____	_____	19.	Assist the client into clean clothes.
_____	_____	_____	20.	Remove the basin, dirty linens, and the other equipment away from the bed.
_____	_____	_____	21.	Change the bed linens using the procedure for making an occupied bed.
_____	_____	_____	22.	Leave the client in a comfortable position. After all the activities, the client may require a rest period.
_____	_____	_____	23.	Wash your hands.
_____	_____	_____	24.	Document procedure and time, observations, and client's reaction.

All items must be successfully completed in this skill. The practice column is for student/partner use. The instructor will check, date, and initial the other two columns.

Practice	Satisfactory	Unsatisfactory	Procedural Steps
_____	_____	_____	1. Wash hands.
_____	_____	_____	2. Assemble supplies: small towel lotion
_____	_____	_____	3. Provide privacy for the client.
_____	_____	_____	4. Position client on back or side.
_____	_____	_____	5. Place small amount of lotion on your hands. Rub together to warm the lotion.
_____	_____	_____	6. Begin by starting at the base of the spine; rub toward the neck in the center of the back. Use both hands in one long stroke.
_____	_____	_____	7. When reaching the neck, continue back down the sides of the back. When reaching the base of the spine, rub up the center again. Repeat several times.
_____	_____	_____	8. If necessary, add more lotion and use a spiral motion for several minutes.
_____	_____	_____	9. Remove excess lotion with small towel. Reposition client.
_____	_____	_____	10. Wash hands and return supplies to proper place.
_____	_____	_____	11. Record and report any sign of skin irritation.

All items must be successfully completed in this skill. The practice column is for student/partner use. The instructor will check, date, and initial the other two columns.

Practice	*Satisfactory*	*Unsatisfactory*		*Procedural Steps*
_____	_____	_____	1.	Assemble supplies: soap basin gloves water washcloths and towel
_____	_____	_____	2.	Wash your hands and apply gloves.
_____	_____	_____	3.	Tell client what you plan to do.
_____	_____	_____	4.	Position client on back and place sheet or thin cotton blanket over client.
_____	_____	_____	5.	Position towel under client's buttocks.
_____	_____	_____	6.	Wet washcloth with soap and water. Help the client flex her knees and spread her legs if able.
_____	_____	_____	7.	Separate the vulva. Clean downward from front to back with one stroke first the inner labia and then rinse. Repeat with outer labia. Repeat on other side. Dry with the towel.
_____	_____	_____	8.	Help the client lower her legs and turn onto her side away from you.
_____	_____	_____	9.	Apply soap to washcloth.
_____	_____	_____	10.	Clean the rectal area by cleaning from the vagina to the anus with one stroke. Rinse washcloth and repeat until area is clean.
_____	_____	_____	11.	Pat the area dry with towel.
_____	_____	_____	12.	Cover client with sheet or blanket and make her comfortable.
_____	_____	_____	13.	Remove basin and supplies from bedside.
_____	_____	_____	14.	Remove your gloves and wash your hands.
_____	_____	_____	15.	Document procedure completed, observations, time, and client's reactions.

PROCEDURE 25:   GIVING MALE PERINEAL CARE

All items must be successfully completed in this skill. The practice column is for student/partner use. The instructor will check, date, and initial the other two columns.

Practice	*Satisfactory*	*Unsatisfactory*	*Procedural Steps*
_____	_____	_____	1. Repeat steps 1 through 6 as for female perineal care.
_____	_____	_____	2. Grasp penis gently with gloved hand. Clean the tip of the penis using gentle circular motion. You will need to pull back the foreskin if the man is uncircumcised. Start at the urinary meatus and work outward. Rinse the area well and dry. Return the foreskin to its original position.
_____	_____	_____	3. Clean the remaining portion of the penis with firm downward strokes. Rinse well.
_____	_____	_____	4. Wash the scrotum and pat dry.
_____	_____	_____	5. Turn client to side and clean rectal area in the same way as for the female.
_____	_____	_____	6. Follow steps 11 through 15 as for female perineal care.

All items must be successfully completed in this skill. The practice column is for student/partner use. The instructor will check, date, and initial the other two columns.

Assistive Devices to Prevent Pressure Sores

Practice	*Satisfactory*	*Unsatisfactory*	*Procedural Steps*
_____	_____	_____	1. Air mattress—This is a mattress filled with air. This works by continuously changing the pressure areas on the client's back. One can improvise an air mattress designed for camping instead of buying a medical air mattress.
_____	_____	_____	2. Egg crate mattress—This is a mattress made of foam rubber that is molded like an egg crate. They are inexpensive, but effective in reducing pressure on the skin. You can also purchase one the size of a seat for the client to sit on during the day when up in a chair.
_____	_____	_____	3. Water mattress—This is similar to a regular water mattress used in homes. This mattress is effective in reducing pressure on the skin, but causes problems when transferring clients in and out of bed.
_____	_____	_____	4. Gel foam cushion—This is a special cushion filled with a special solution or gel. This style of cushion is effective in the prevention of pressure sores for a client who sits in a wheelchair for long periods of time.
_____	_____	_____	5. Sheepskin or lamb's wool pads or elbow or heel pads—Lamb's wool pads prevent pressure sores by acting as a barrier between the client's skin and the sheets.
_____	_____	_____	6. Bed cradle—This is a device to keep linens off the client's legs and feet. In the home a client may substitute a box or other device to keep linens off the legs and feet

Practice	Satisfactory	Unsatisfactory		Procedural Steps
				Special Care to Prevent Pressure Sores
_____	_____	_____	1.	Change client's position at least every 2 hours to reduce pressure on any one area.
_____	_____	_____	2.	As quickly as possible, remove feces, urine, or moisture of any kind that might be irritating the skin.
_____	_____	_____	3.	Encourage clients who sit in chairs or wheelchairs to raise themselves or change position every 15 minutes to relieve pressure.
_____	_____	_____	4.	Encourage client to eat a high protein diet if allowed and drink adequate fluids.
_____	_____	_____	5.	Keep bed linens clean, dry, and wrinkle free.
_____	_____	_____	6.	When bathing clients use soap sparingly because soap dries skin. Keep skin well lubricated.
_____	_____	_____	7.	Watch for skin irritation when applying braces and splints.
_____	_____	_____	8.	At the first sign of a reddened area, gently massage area around the reddened area. Report your observations to the nurse supervisor.

All items must be successfully completed in this skill. The practice column is for student/partner use. The instructor will check, date, and initial the other two columns.

Practice	Satisfactory	Unsatisfactory	Procedural Steps
_____	_____	_____	1. Assemble needed equipment and supplies: toothbrush / toothpaste / gloves / glass of water / towel / small bowl or basin or emesis basin / mouthwash if available / tissues or damp washcloth
_____	_____	_____	2. Wash your hands and apply gloves.
_____	_____	_____	3. Tell client what you plan to do and position the client in a sitting position (if allowed).
_____	_____	_____	4. Place a towel over the client's chest and under the chin.
_____	_____	_____	5. Moisten toothbrush and apply toothpaste.
_____	_____	_____	6. Let client brush teeth, if able. If not, carefully brush the client's teeth.
_____	_____	_____	7. Give the client a glass of water; be sure client rinses mouth well. Hold the basin underneath the client's chin and have client return the fluid. If mouthwash is available, have client rinse mouth with the mouthwash.
_____	_____	_____	8. Give the client a moistened washcloth to wipe mouth.
_____	_____	_____	9. Reposition client.
_____	_____	_____	10. Clean and replace equipment.
_____	_____	_____	11. Remove gloves and wash hands.
_____	_____	_____	12. Document procedure completed and time, any observations and client's reaction.

PROCEDURE 28:   CARING FOR DENTURES

All items must be successfully completed in this skill. The practice column is for student/partner use. The instructor will check, date, and initial the other two columns.

Practice	Satisfactory	Unsatisfactory		Procedural Steps
_____	_____	_____	1.	Assemble the needed supplies:
				denture cup or two small containers lined with gauze or washcloth for padding
				toothbrush and toothpaste
				mouthwash with small cup
				small towel and dampened washcloth
				gloves
_____	_____	_____	2.	Wash your hands and apply gloves.
_____	_____	_____	3.	Tell client what you plan to do.
_____	_____	_____	4.	Ask client to remove dentures, helping if needed. Place dentures in padded container or denture cup. Be very careful in handling client's dentures. They may become slippery to hold.
_____	_____	_____	5.	Place approximately 2 to 3 inches of water and a small paper towel in bottom of sink. This will protect the dentures in case they are dropped. Turn on cold water and brush all surfaces of the upper and lower plate. Rinse denture cup and place fresh gauze squares into bottom. Place dentures in cup and take to client's bedside.
_____	_____	_____	6.	Assist client to rinse mouth with mouthwash.
_____	_____	_____	7.	A soft toothbrush or other type of applicator may be used to clean the mouth while dentures are out. This is a good time to observe the inside of the client's mouth for signs of irritation or soreness.
_____	_____	_____	8.	Have client, if capable, insert clean dentures into mouth.
_____	_____	_____	9.	Clean and replace equipment.
_____	_____	_____	10.	Remove gloves and wash hands.
_____	_____	_____	11.	Document procedure completed and time, observations, and client's reaction.

All items must be successfully completed in this skill. The practice column is for student/partner use. The instructor will check, date, and initial the other two columns.

Practice	Satisfactory	Unsatisfactory	Procedural Steps
_____	_____	_____	1. Wash hands and apply gloves.
_____	_____	_____	2. Ask client if he wants a shave.
_____	_____	_____	3. Assemble needed supplies. If possible have client shave in bathroom by the mirror.
			gloves
			razor and shaving cream
			basin of hot water
			washcloth and towel
			aftershave lotion (optional)
_____	_____	_____	4. Position client in sitting position and place towel under chin and across his chest.
_____	_____	_____	5. Wet client's face with shaving cream. With one hand pull the skin tight above area to be shaved. With razor in other hand, gently take short, even strokes. Shave in the direction the hair grows. If client is capable, let him do as much as possible.
_____	_____	_____	6. Rinse the razor frequently. After shave is completed, place used uncapped razor in "sharps" containers.
_____	_____	_____	7. Change water in basin when shave is completed. Rinse the client's face in clear warm water and pat dry.
_____	_____	_____	8. If desired, apply aftershave lotion. Remove gloves.
_____	_____	_____	9. Return equipment and supplies, clean and rinse basin, dry and store.
_____	_____	_____	10. Reposition client.
_____	_____	_____	11. Wash hands.
_____	_____	_____	12. Document completion of procedure and time, observations, and client's reaction.

PROCEDURE 30: DRESSING AND UNDRESSING THE CLIENT

All items must be successfully completed in this skill. The practice column is for student/partner use. The instructor will check, date, and initial the other two columns.

Practice	*Satisfactory*	*Unsatisfactory*	*Procedural Steps*
_____	_____	_____	1. Wash your hands and tell client what you plan to do.
_____	_____	_____	2. Assemble clean clothing: undergarments outergarments—let client select if possible stockings and shoes
_____	_____	_____	3. If client is able, help the client to sit at the edge of the bed and dangle the legs. If the client is too weak to sit up, have client lie flat on the bed. Place a sheet or robe over client to avoid embarrassing or chilling the client.
_____	_____	_____	4. Assist the client to put on undergarments. If client has weak leg, place weak leg in first, then the other leg. Then put on outergarments in the same manner. If client can stand, pull the pants or slacks up to the waist. If the client must remain on the bed, ask the client to press the heels into the bed and raise the buttocks. While the client is in this position, quickly slide the pants or slacks up to the waist. Assist the client as necessary. Slacks with elastic waist are preferred as they go on easier than pants with zippers and buttons. Cotton jogging suits are becoming a very popular option for the disabled or elderly clients. They are warm, easy to get off and on, and attractive. They also launder easily.
_____	_____	_____	5. To dress the client in a shirt, slip, or dress, help the client place the weak arm into the sleeve first, then the strong arm. If dress or shirt needs to go over head, help client place both arms into armholes and then slip the neck of the garment over the client's head.

Practice	Satisfactory	Unsatisfactory		Procedural Steps
_____	_____	_____	6.	To put on socks or stockings, turn each sock down to the toe end. Slide client's toe into place and, with one arm on each side of leg, pull the sock or stocking up. Make sure socks are smooth over the feet and legs. Put on shoes if the client is to remain out of bed. Let client assist as much as possible.
_____	_____	_____	7.	To undress the client, simply reverse the instruction for dressing. If the client has a weak arm or leg, undress the weak limb last.
_____	_____	_____	8.	Wash hands.

PROCEDURE 31:   APPLYING ELASTICIZED STOCKINGS

All items must be successfully completed in this skill. The practice column is for student/partner use. The instructor will check, date, and initial the other two columns.

Practice	Satisfactory	Unsatisfactory	Procedural Steps
_____	_____	_____	1. Wash your hands
_____	_____	_____	2. Tell client what you plan to do.
_____	_____	_____	3. With client lying down, expose one leg at a time.
_____	_____	_____	4. Turn stocking inside out to heel by placing your hand inside stocking and grasping heel. Position stocking over foot and heel of client, making sure the heel is properly placed. Continue to pull the remaining part of the hose upward over the client's leg.
_____	_____	_____	5. Check to be sure stocking is applied evenly and smoothly and there are no wrinkles.
_____	_____	_____	6. Repeat procedure on opposite leg.
_____	_____	_____	7. Wash your hands.
_____	_____	_____	8. Document time and completion of the procedure and client's reaction.

All items must be successfully completed in this skill. The practice column is for student/partner use. The instructor will check, date, and initial the other two columns.

Practice	Satisfactory	Unsatisfactory	Procedural Steps
_____	_____	_____	1. Strip bed of dirty linens and place in laundry.
_____	_____	_____	2. Wash hands.
_____	_____	_____	3. Assemble clean linens: top sheet and fitted bottom sheet, if available pillow cases mattress pad, bedspread, and blankets if needed
_____	_____	_____	4. Place mattress pad on bed and then put clean fitted sheet or flat sheet on bed. If flat sheet is being used, unfold the sheet with the long fold at the center of the bed. Place lower hemline even with the bottom of the mattress.
_____	_____	_____	5. Open sheet gently; do not shake. Starting at the head of the bed, miter the corner and tuck in that side of the sheet. A great deal of time is saved by working on only one side of the bed at a time. Sizes of bedrooms differ greatly in client's homes; you will need to adjust this procedure to your client's bed placement in the home.
_____	_____	_____	6. Place top sheet over the bottom sheet wrong side up. Place hem even with the top edge of the mattress. Place the center fold at the center of the bed. Tuck in top sheet at foot of bed and make a mitered corner. (**Note:** The top sheet, blanket, and spread, if used, may be tucked under the mattress at the same time.)
_____	_____	_____	7. Place the blanket back on the bed. Put the top edge 12 inches from the top of the mattress. Place bedspread on the bed.

Practice	Satisfactory	Unsatisfactory		Procedural Steps
_____	_____	_____	8.	Tuck the blanket and top sheet under the bottom of the mattress at the foot end of the bed. Miter the corner. Fold top sheet over the top edge of the bed.
_____	_____	_____	9.	Walk over to opposite side of bed and make remaining part of the bed.
_____	_____	_____	10.	Put pillowcases on pillows.
_____	_____	_____	11.	Wash your hands.
_____	_____	_____	12.	Document task completed.

All items must be successfully completed in this skill. The practice column is for student/partner use. The instructor will check, date, and initial the other two columns.

Practice	Satisfactory	Unsatisfactory	Procedural Steps
_____	_____	_____	1. Wash your hands.
_____	_____	_____	2. Assemble clean linens: flat sheet and fitted bottom (if available) extra flat sheet or drawsheet if used by client pillow cases large plastic bag (for soiled linens)
_____	_____	_____	3. Tell client what you plan to do and provide for the client's privacy by closing the bedroom door.
_____	_____	_____	4. Place clean linen on a clean chair or table in room in the order you plan to use them.
_____	_____	_____	5. Loosen bedding from under mattress by lifting mattress with one hand as you pull out bedding with the other hand.
_____	_____	_____	6. Remove top covers one at a time, folding each to the foot of the bed.
_____	_____	_____	7. Leave top sheet covering the client to prevent chilling and afford privacy.
_____	_____	_____	8. Place two straight chairs against one side of the bed. This helps protect the client from falling out of bed. If the bed has side rails this is not necessary. Simply raise the side rail on the opposite side of the bed.
_____	_____	_____	9. Assist the client to turn on the side facing the chairs or side rail. Assist the client to move near the edge of the bed by the chairs. Stand at the other side of the bed.
_____	_____	_____	10. Roll or fanfold (fold in pleats) the soiled bottom sheet to the center of the bed beside the client's back.
_____	_____	_____	11. Fold the clean bottom sheet lengthwise and place the fold at the center of the bed. Fanfold half the clean sheet next to the soiled sheet. Tuck the other half under the mattress. Make a mitered corner at the top. Tuck from the top or head of bed and move toward the foot of the bed.

Practice	Satisfactory	Unsatisfactory		Procedural Steps
_____	_____	_____	12.	Help client turn toward you onto the clean sheet. Bring the chairs to the other side of the bed for the client's protection (or raise the side rail).
_____	_____	_____	13.	Go to the other side and remove soiled sheet. Place dirty linen into large plastic bag.
_____	_____	_____	14.	Pull clean sheet across bed and tuck under mattress. Miter corner at top and tuck along side from head to foot of bed. Make certain the sheet is tight and wrinkle free.
_____	_____	_____	15.	Turn client onto the back in center of the bed. Place clean top sheet over the soiled top sheet. Slide the soiled sheet out from under the clean sheet. Have client hold fresh top sheet in place.
_____	_____	_____	16.	Place soiled sheet in large plastic bag.
_____	_____	_____	17.	Unfold blankets and place over top sheet.
_____	_____	_____	18.	Tuck in the bottoms of the sheet, blanket, and bedspread at the foot of the bed. Miter the two corners; leave extra room for foot and toe movement.
_____	_____	_____	19.	Change the pillow cases and replace pillows under client's head. Put soiled cases in large plastic bag.
_____	_____	_____	20.	Be sure client is comfortable and that the room is neat. Remove soiled linens from room.
_____	_____	_____	21.	Wash your hands.
_____	_____	_____	22.	Document procedure completed.

PROCEDURE 34: GIVING NAIL CARE

All items must be successfully completed in this skill. The practice column is for student/partner use. The instructor will check, date, and initial the other two columns.

Practice	Satisfactory	Unsatisfactory	Procedural Steps
_____	_____	_____	1. Assemble supplies: soap, water, and basin nail brush towel and lotion, preferably lanolin lotion small scissors or clippers emery board or nail file
_____	_____	_____	2. Wash your hands.
_____	_____	_____	3. Tell client what you plan to do.
_____	_____	_____	4. Soak toenails or fingernails in soap and water for 10 minutes.
_____	_____	_____	5. Brush nails with nail brush. Clean under nails. Rinse well. Dry hands and nails.
_____	_____	_____	6. Wear gloves if clipping nails/toenails.
_____	_____	_____	7. If nails are too long, make a straight cut for toenails and a curve cut for fingernails. Check to make sure that you are allowed to cut nails.
_____	_____	_____	8. Use file or emery board and smooth edges of nails.
_____	_____	_____	9. Massage lotion on the hands or feet.
_____	_____	_____	10. If you accidently cut a client's skin while cutting nails, remember to use universal precautions. Report the cut to your supervisor.
_____	_____	_____	11. Clean the basin, brush, and scissors or clippers. Return equipment to proper place.
_____	_____	_____	12. Wash your hands.
_____	_____	_____	13. Document procedure, any observations, and client's reaction.

PROCEDURE 35:   SHAMPOOING THE CLIENT'S HAIR IN BED

All items must be successfully completed in this skill. The practice column is for student/partner use. The instructor will check, date, and initial the other two columns.

Practice	*Satisfactory*	*Unsatisfactory*	*Procedural Steps*
_____	_____	_____	1. Assemble equipment: shampoo and hair conditioner or rinse (optional) 3 or 4 towels large plastic garbage bags or rubber sheet large empty container or large wastepaper basket or bucket large pitcher for warm water comb and brush disposable gloves newspapers
_____	_____	_____	2. Wash your hands. If client has sores or lesions of the scalp, wear gloves.
_____	_____	_____	3. Tell client what you plan to do.
_____	_____	_____	4. Position client so that the head rests over the edge of the bed. The back and shoulders should rest on the edge. (Your instructor will demonstrate this procedure.)
_____	_____	_____	5. Loosen clothing from around client's neck. Roll a towel to be placed around neck.
_____	_____	_____	6. Spread a newspaper on a chair or on the floor and set large empty bucket or container on the newspaper. Move the chair with the basin to a position beneath the head of the client.
_____	_____	_____	7. Slide a plastic bag or sheet under the client's shoulders. Let the other end of the plastic fall into the basin. This allows the water to go from the head into the catch basin or bucket.
_____	_____	_____	8. With pitcher full of warm water, wet the client's hair.

Practice	Satisfactory	Unsatisfactory	Procedural Steps
_____	_____	_____	9. Apply shampoo to the head, lather well, and massage scalp with your knuckles. If nonprescription medicated shampoo is ordered, please follow any special instructions on label.
_____	_____	_____	10. Rinse hair with water thoroughly, making sure to remove all traces of shampoo.
_____	_____	_____	11. If necessary, reapply shampoo, lather well, and rinse thoroughly.
_____	_____	_____	12. Apply hair conditioner or rinse. Follow directions on the bottle, as some need to be diluted and others do not.
_____	_____	_____	13. Dry client's hair with large towel. Comb and brush hair. If female, you may need to set hair on rollers. If hair dryer is available, blow dry hair gently.
_____	_____	_____	14. Return equipment to proper storage area.
_____	_____	_____	15. Wash hands.
_____	_____	_____	16. Document procedure completed, your observations, and client's reaction.

PROCEDURE 36: ASSISTING THE CLIENT WITH SELF-ADMINISTERED MEDICATIONS

All items must be successfully completed in this skill. The practice column is for student/partner use. The instructor will check, date, and initial the other two columns.

Practice	*Satisfactory*	*Unsatisfactory*	*Procedural Steps*
_____	_____	_____	1. Have the nurse supervisor or pharmacist prepare a list of medications prescribed and the time they are to be given. Some medications are given 3 times a day (tid), usually before (ac) or after (pc) each meal. Others may be ordered 4 times a day (qid) or every 6 hours (q6h). A medication taken every 6 hours could be given at 6 AM, noon, 6 PM, and midnight. The pharmacist usually informs the client at which times the medications should be taken.
_____	_____	_____	2. The nurse supervisor will set a schedule to be followed daily. After each medication has been taken, check it off. This informs both the aide and the client that the medicine has been taken. Refer to the schedule and remind the client when medicine is due. Your nurse supervisor may prepare your client's medication in special containers that have all the medication needed for a specific time.
_____	_____	_____	3. Check with the client each time to make sure the medicine is the correct one listed on the schedule.
_____	_____	_____	4. Make sure the correct method of taking the medication is followed. For example, some medicines are taken with juice or milk instead of water. Others are taken on an empty stomach, others with food.
_____	_____	_____	5. Certain medications such as nitroglycerin tablets must be within the client's reach at all times. When the client has chest pain, the client needs to place these tablets under the tongue immediately.
_____	_____	_____	6. Be sure sleeping and pain medication bottles are kept in a safe place after each use. They should only be taken as often as the doctor has ordered.

Practice	*Satisfactory*	*Unsatisfactory*		*Procedural Steps*
_____	_____	_____	7.	Review the times with the client when the prescribed medications are to be taken. Leave the medication within easy reach of the client. Remind the client to take the nighttime dose in a well-lit room.
_____	_____	_____	8.	If the client has questions about the medications, encourage the client to ask the pharmacist, nurse supervisor, or doctor. The client should be knowledgeable about medications that he or she is taking.
_____	_____	_____	9.	As a home health aide, you are not allowed to pour the client's medication from the bottle; the client needs to do this himself/herself.

PROCEDURE 37:   INSERTING A HEARING AID

All items must be successfully completed in this skill. The practice column is for student/partner use. The instructor will check, date, and initial the other two columns.

Practice	*Satisfactory*	*Unsatisfactory*	*Procedural Steps*
_____	_____	_____	1. Wash your hands.
_____	_____	_____	2. Check hearing aid appliance to see that the batteries are working and tubing is not cracked.
_____	_____	_____	3. Tell the client what you plan to do. You may need to use gestures because client may not be able to hear spoken words.
_____	_____	_____	4. Check inside of client's ear for wax buildup or any other abnormalities.
_____	_____	_____	5. Check to make sure the hearing aid is off or the volume is turned to its lowest level.
_____	_____	_____	6. Handle the hearing aid very carefully. Do not drop it or allow it to get wet. Store in a safe area when client is not wearing it. Be sure hearing aid is clean before giving it to client. Follow manufacturer's directions in cleaning your client's hearing aid.
_____	_____	_____	7. Assist the client in inserting the earmold in the ear canal.

Alternate Actions

_____	_____	_____	8. Place the hearing aid over the client's ear, allowing the earmold to hang free.
_____	_____	_____	9. Adjust the hearing aid behind the client's ear.
_____	_____	_____	10. Grasp the earmold and gently insert the tapered end into the ear canal.
_____	_____	_____	11. Gently twist the earmold into the curve of the ear, pushing upward and inward on the bottom of the earmold, while pulling on the ear lobe with the other hand.
_____	_____	_____	12. Let client turn on switch and adjust volume.
_____	_____	_____	13. Wash hands.

PROCEDURE 38:   CARING FOR AN ARTIFICIAL EYE

All items must be successfully completed in this skill. The practice column is for student/partner use. The instructor will check, date, and initial the other two columns.

Practice	Satisfactory	Unsatisfactory	Procedural Steps
_____	_____	_____	1. Assemble equipment : eyecup with gauze square (not cotton filled) cleansing solution, if ordered washcloth and basin of lukewarm water gloves cotton balls small plastic bag for wastes
_____	_____	_____	2. Wash hands and apply gloves.
_____	_____	_____	3. Tell client what you plan to do.
_____	_____	_____	4. Have client lie down if possible. Position yourself and equipment to be on the same side as the client's artificial eye.
_____	_____	_____	5. With moistened cotton balls clean the outside of the eye from the nose to the outside of the face. Stroke once only with each cotton ball.
_____	_____	_____	6. Remove artificial eye by depressing lower eyelid with your thumb while lifting upper lid with your index finger. If client can remove artificial eye, let the client do it. Carefully take eye and place in gauze lined eyecup. Place eyecup in a very safe place nearby while you clean the outside of the eye socket.
_____	_____	_____	7. Clean eye socket using warm water and cotton balls. Pat area around eye dry. Observe area for signs of irritation or infection.
_____	_____	_____	8. Carry eyecup to bathroom. Place washcloth in bottom of sink, as a precaution against breakage. Remove eye from eyecup and gently wash in sink. Remove all secretions on outside of the eye. Do not use any cleaner on eye unless specifically ordered.

Practice	Satisfactory	Unsatisfactory	Procedural Steps
_____	_____	_____	9. Place clean gauze in bottom of eyecup and return to client. Assist the client to insert eye into socket. If eye is moist, it will slide in easier. You may need to depress the lower eyelid and slip gently over the eye as it slips into the socket.
_____	_____	_____	10. If client does not wish to have eye inserted into socket right away, the eye needs to be stored in water in the eyecup.
_____	_____	_____	11. Return equipment and wastes to correct areas.
_____	_____	_____	12. If client wears glasses, clean the glasses with a cleaning solution, rinse with clear water, and dry with tissues. Handle the glasses only by the frame. Return glasses to client or place in case.
_____	_____	_____	13. Remove gloves and wash hands.
_____	_____	_____	14. Document procedure completion, your observations, and client's reaction.

PROCEDURE 39:   FEEDING THE CLIENT

All items must be successfully completed in this skill. The practice column is for student/partner use. The instructor will check, date, and initial the other two columns.

Practice	Satisfactory	Unsatisfactory		Procedural Steps
_____	_____	_____	1.	Wash your hands.
_____	_____	_____	2.	Prepare the client to eat. Wash the client's face and hands. Position client in sitting position in bed or sitting up in a chair. Make environment as pleasant as possible. If necessary do mouth care before to increase the client's desire to eat. Place large napkin over client's chest.
_____	_____	_____	3.	Bring food to client. Tell client what foods you prepared.
_____	_____	_____	4.	How you feed or assist your client depends on the handicap or physical problem the client has. If the client is blind, you need to tell the client where each food is on the plate in relation to a clock. If the client has use of only one hand, a suction plate or plate guard may be used. If the client cannot chew food, the food will need to be soft in consistency. **Caution:** The client should never be given cause to be embarrassed because of any physical disability.
_____	_____	_____	5.	Ask the client which food is desired first. (Getting the client's cooperation and participation is important.)
_____	_____	_____	6.	If the client must be fed by the aide, remember:

- Check to see if dentures are in place.

- Feed slowly; let the client set the pace. Thermal bowls and cups will assist in keeping foods at proper temperature.

- Feed small amounts of food at a time.

- Make sure the consistency of the food is appropriate.

- Do not use a syringe to feed the client. A child's feeder cup or plastic glass works well in this situation.

- If possible, have client hold finger foods or bread.

PROCEDURE 40: MEASURING AND RECORDING FLUID INTAKE AND OUTPUT

All items must be successfully completed in this skill. The practice column is for student/partner use. The instructor will check, date, and initial the other two columns.

Practice	*Satisfactory*	*Unsatisfactory*	*Procedural Steps*
_____	_____	_____	1. Assemble supplies: measuring cup or container for intake large measuring container for output
_____	_____	_____	2. Wash hands and apply gloves if measuring output.
_____	_____	_____	3. Measure and record all liquids taken by the client. This includes all fluids taken with meals and between meals: coffee, milk, fruit juices, beer, and water. Liquids are recorded in cubic centimeters, abbreviated cc. You need to remember that 30 cc equals 1 ounce. Example: If a client drank a can of pop that is 12 ounces, you need to multiply 12 by 30, which equals 360 cc.
_____	_____	_____	4. Ask the client to use a urinal or bedpan for all voiding. If the client can use the toilet, a special plastic hat can be placed in the toilet to collect the urine. All urine must be collected so that it can be measured.
_____	_____	_____	5. Pour urine from bedpan or urinal into a measuring device. Record the amount. Always record output in cc.
_____	_____	_____	6. Be sure to explain to the client how to keep exact records. The client will need to record the fluids at times when the aide is off duty.
_____	_____	_____	7. Clean equipment after each use.
_____	_____	_____	8. Remove gloves and wash hands.
_____	_____	_____	9. Document findings.

PROCEDURE 41:   GIVING AND EMPTYING THE BEDPAN

All items must be successfully completed in this skill. The practice column is for student/partner use. The instructor will check, date, and initial the other two columns.

Practice	Satisfactory	Unsatisfactory	Procedural Steps
_____	_____	_____	1. Assemble equipment and supplies needed: bedpan and bedpan cover toilet tissue moistened washcloth
_____	_____	_____	2. Wash hands and apply gloves.
_____	_____	_____	3. Tell client what you plan to do.
_____	_____	_____	4. If a metal bedpan is used, first warm it by running hot water over the rim. Dry the rim and sprinkle it with powder if available. The powder prevents the client's buttocks from sticking to the bedpan.
_____	_____	_____	5. Place bedpan near the bed. Put toilet tissue near the client's hand.
_____	_____	_____	6. Fold top blanket and sheet at an angle. Remove the client's bottom clothing.
_____	_____	_____	7. To raise the buttocks, have the client bend knees and push on the heels. As the client lifts, place your hand under the small of the client's back. The aide holds the bedpan in place when the client is lying on his/her backside and then turns the client.
_____	_____	_____	8. Lift gently and slowly with one hand. Slide the bedpan under the hips with the other hand. The client's buttocks should rest on the rounded shelf of the bedpan. The narrow end should face the foot of the bed. If the client cannot assist, turn the client to one side and position the bedpan over the buttocks. Roll the client onto the bedpan. Make sure the client's head is elevated.
_____	_____	_____	9. Pull sheet over the client for added privacy. Make sure the client is as comfortable as possible. An extra pillow under the head may be used.
_____	_____	_____	10. While client is using the bedpan, the aide can be moistening the washcloth.

Practice	Satisfactory	Unsatisfactory	Procedural Steps
_____	_____	_____	11. Remove the bedpan when the client is finished using it. Do not leave the client sitting on the bedpan for longer than 15 minutes. Remove the bedpan by having the client bend the knees and push on the heels. Place one hand under small of client's back and lift. Remove the bedpan with the other hand.
_____	_____	_____	12. If possible, have clients wipe. If they are not able to do this, the aide must wipe the client. Discard tissues in the bedpan.
_____	_____	_____	13. Replace the client's clothing. Give client washcloth to wipe hands.
_____	_____	_____	14. Take bedpan to toilet, observe contents and measure if necessary. Empty contents into toilet. Flush. Fill bedpan with cold water and empty. Clean bedpan by using warm soapy water and the toilet brush. Empty water into toilet and rinse bedpan. Dry well.
_____	_____	_____	15. Return bedpan to proper storage area.
_____	_____	_____	16. Remove gloves and wash hands.
_____	_____	_____	17. Record amount of urine; color, amount, and consistency of stool.

PROCEDURE 42:   GIVING AND EMPTYING THE URINAL

All items must be successfully completed in this skill. The practice column is for student/partner use. The instructor will check, date, and initial the other two columns.

Practice	Satisfactory	Unsatisfactory	Procedural Steps
_____	_____	_____	1. Wash your hands and apply gloves.
_____	_____	_____	2. Lift the top bedcovers and place the urinal under the covers so that the client can grasp the handle. If he cannot do this, you must place the urinal in position and ensure the penis is placed in the opening of the urinal. If possible, assist the client to stand when using the urinal.
_____	_____	_____	3. Remove gloves and dispose of them properly. Leave the client alone if possible. You may give the client a bell to ring when he is done.
_____	_____	_____	4. Put on gloves and remove urinal once client is done using it.
_____	_____	_____	5. Take the urinal to the bathroom and observe contents. Measure if required. Empty the urinal. Rinse with cold water and clean with soapy water. Rinse with disinfectant or water, dry, store properly.
_____	_____	_____	6. Remove gloves and wash hands.
_____	_____	_____	7. Record amount and color of urine, as required.

All items must be successfully completed in this skill. The practice column is for student/partner use. The instructor will check, date, and initial the other two columns.

Practice	*Satisfactory*	*Unsatisfactory*	*Procedural Steps*
_____	_____	_____	1. Assemble needed supplies: sterile urine specimen container with completed label plastic or zip-lock bag and paper bag gloves clean bedpan or urinal antiseptic soaked wipes
_____	_____	_____	2. Wash hands and apply gloves.
_____	_____	_____	3. Inform client of what you plan to do.
_____	_____	_____	4. Wash the client's genital area or have the client do so, if able. It is especially important for the urinary opening to be cleansed.
_____	_____	_____	5. Give the client a labeled specimen container.
_____	_____	_____	6. Explain the procedure to the client.
_____	_____	_____	7. Have the client begin to void into the bedpan, urinal, or toilet. After a small amount of urine has been voided, have the client catch some of the urine in midstream in the sterile specimen container. You will only need 2 ounces or 60 cc. After the specimen has been collected, the client can resume voiding into the bedpan, urinal, or toilet.
_____	_____	_____	8. Immediately place the sterile cap on the specimen container so the specimen will not become contaminated.
_____	_____	_____	9. Remove bedpan and wipe client.
_____	_____	_____	10. Place labeled specimen container inside a plastic bag or zip-lock bag, then put this bag inside a paper bag with completed label.
_____	_____	_____	11. Remove gloves and wash hands.
_____	_____	_____	12. Place specimen bag in refrigerator until time to take to local laboratory.
_____	_____	_____	13. Document time of collection and type of specimen.

All items must be successfully completed in this skill. The practice column is for student/partner use. The instructor will check, date, and initial the other two columns.

Practice	*Satisfactory*	*Unsatisfactory*	*Procedural Steps*
_____	_____	_____	1. Assemble supplies: gloves antiseptic wipes basin of warm water plastic bag for waste cotton-tipped applicators
_____	_____	_____	2. Wash your hands and apply gloves.
_____	_____	_____	3. Tell client what you plan to do.
_____	_____	_____	4. Position client on his/her back. Expose only a small area where the catheter enters the body. Using soap and warm water or antiseptic wipes, wash area surrounding the catheter.
_____	_____	_____	5. Using antiseptic wipes or gauze pads dipped in warm water, wipe the catheter tube. Make only one stroke with each swab or pad. Discard each wipe after one stroke. Start at the urinary opening and wipe *away* from it. Be careful not to dislodge the catheter. Clean the catheter up to the connection of the drainage tubing.
_____	_____	_____	6. Remove gloves and discard into plastic bag.
_____	_____	_____	7. Check to be sure tubing is coiled on bed and hanging straight down into the drainage container. Check level of urine in the collection bag. Tubing should not be below the collection bag. Do not raise collection bag above the level of the client's bladder.
_____	_____	_____	8. Cover client and discard wastes properly.
_____	_____	_____	9. Wash hands.
_____	_____	_____	10. Document procedure and time, your observations, and client's reaction.

PROCEDURE 45: CONNECTING THE LEG BAG

All items must be successfully completed in this skill. The practice column is for student/partner use. The instructor will check, date, and initial the other two columns.

Practice	Satisfactory	Unsatisfactory		Procedural Steps
_____	_____	_____	1.	Assemble needed equipment: leg bag, alcohol wipes, paper towels, gloves
_____	_____	_____	2.	Wash your hands and apply gloves.
_____	_____	_____	3.	Tell client what you plan to do.
_____	_____	_____	4.	Place paper towel underneath catheter connection area.
_____	_____	_____	5.	Use alcohol to disinfect area to be disconnected.
_____	_____	_____	6.	Disconnect catheter from tubing. Wipe end of catheter with alcohol. Remove cap from end of leg bag and connect leg bag to catheter. Place cap on end of closed drainage system.
_____	_____	_____	7.	Attach leg straps and bag to leg of client. Check to see if the part marked "top" of bag is in the correct position.
_____	_____	_____	8.	Empty and measure urine from bedside collection bag.
_____	_____	_____	9.	Remove gloves and wash hands.
_____	_____	_____	10.	Document procedure completed.

All items must be successfully completed in this skill. The practice column is for student/partner use. The instructor will check, date, and initial the other two columns.

Practice	Satisfactory	Unsatisfactory	Procedural Steps
_____	_____	_____	1. Assemble equipment: gloves, alcohol wipes, measuring device, paper towel
_____	_____	_____	2. Wash hands and apply gloves.
_____	_____	_____	3. Tell client what you plan to do.
_____	_____	_____	4. Place paper towel and measuring device on floor below drainage bag.
_____	_____	_____	5. Open drain or spout and allow the urine to drain into measuring device. Do not allow the tip of tubing to touch sides of the measuring device.
_____	_____	_____	6. Close the drain and wipe it with the alcohol wipe. Replace it in the holder on the bag.
_____	_____	_____	7. Note the amount and color of urine. Empty urine into toilet. Wash and rinse measuring device.
_____	_____	_____	8. Remove gloves and wash hands.
_____	_____	_____	9. Document amount.

PROCEDURE 47: RETRAINING THE BLADDER

All items must be successfully completed in this skill. The practice column is for student/partner use. The instructor will check, date, and initial the other two columns.

Practice	*Satisfactory*	*Unsatisfactory*	*Procedural Steps*
_____	_____	_____	1. A health care team assesses prior habits of a client. If a client normally voids about every 3–4 hours, this would be important to know in planning the client's retraining program
_____	_____	_____	2. A plan is designed and implemented. Important elements of the plan are: • good intake of fluids • toileting client at regular intervals • easy on-easy off clothing so that no "accidents" occur as a result of the clothing • praise by the aide when progress is made by the client • privacy for voiding
_____	_____	_____	3. Follow the bladder retraining program developed. If plan appears to be working, document results. If plan doesn't appear to be working, report this to case manager and other home health care team members as needed.

PROCEDURE 48: COLLECTING A SPUTUM SPECIMEN

All items must be successfully completed in this skill. The practice column is for student/partner use. The instructor will check, date, and initial the other two columns.

Practice	Satisfactory	Unsatisfactory	Procedural Steps
_____	_____	_____	1. Assemble supplies: specimen container, cover with label completed tissues gloves moisture-proof plastic bag mask (optional)
_____	_____	_____	2. Wash hands and apply gloves. Wear a mask if client has an infectious disease.
_____	_____	_____	3. Ask client to cough deeply and bring up sputum from the lungs. Have client expectorate (spit) into the container. Collect 1 to 2 tablespoons of sputum unless otherwise directed. Be sure to have client cover mouth with tissue to prevent the spread of infections. If excess sputum contaminates the outside of the container, wipe off right away. Cover specimen container and place in moisture-proof bag.
_____	_____	_____	4. Remove gloves and wash hands.
_____	_____	_____	5. Document collection of sputum and when transported to laboratory.

PROCEDURE 49: TAKING AN ORAL TEMPERATURE

All items must be successfully completed in this skill. The practice column is for student/partner use. The instructor will check, date, and initial the other two columns.

Practice	Satisfactory	Unsatisfactory	Procedural Steps
_____	_____	_____	1. Ask the client not to drink any liquids or smoke 15 minutes before the temperature is taken. Otherwise an inaccurate reading could result.
_____	_____	_____	2. Gather the equipment needed: oral thermometer / tissues / pad and pencil / watch with second hand / alcohol / gloves
_____	_____	_____	3. Wash your hands thoroughly and put on gloves.
_____	_____	_____	4. Ask the client to find a comfortable position, either in a chair or in a bed.
_____	_____	_____	5. Hold thermometer by stem end and read mercury column. It should register 96°F or lower (35.5°C). If it does not, shake down the thermometer with a snap of the wrist. Shake the thermometer down until it reads 94°F (34.4°C).
_____	_____	_____	6. Insert bulb end of thermometer under client's tongue. Slant it toward the side of the mouth. Ask the client to close the mouth and place the thermometer under the tongue.
_____	_____	_____	7. Be sure the client holds the thermometer under the tongue for a minimum of 3 minutes and then remove the thermometer.
_____	_____	_____	8. Gently wipe the thermometer with a tissue from the stem to the bulb end. Discard the contaminated tissue. If using a cover, discard it.

Practice	Satisfactory	Unsatisfactory	Procedural Steps
_____	_____	_____	9. Hold the thermometer at eye level and record the measurement. Normal oral temperature is 98.6°F (37°C). Mark down the time the reading was made and the temperature reading. Report any temperature which reads above 101°F (38°C).
_____	_____	_____	10. Clean the thermometer by washing it with a small amount of soap and cold water. Rinse all soap from the thermometer. A tissue wet in alcohol may also be used to clean the thermometer. Wipe from stem end to the front, bulb end (clean to dirty).
_____	_____	_____	11. The client may have an electric thermometer with a digital readout.
_____	_____	_____	12. Return the thermometer to the proper storage place.
_____	_____	_____	13. Remove gloves and wash your hands after the procedure.

PROCEDURE 50:   TAKING A RECTAL TEMPERATURE

All items must be successfully completed in this skill. The practice column is for student/partner use. The instructor will check, date, and initial the other two columns.

Practice	Satisfactory	Unsatisfactory	Procedural Steps
_____	_____	_____	1. Gather the equipment needed: rectal thermometer lubricant tissues pad and pencil watch with second hand alcohol gloves
_____	_____	_____	2. Wash your hands thoroughly and apply gloves.
_____	_____	_____	3. Tell the client that you plan to take a rectal temperature. Provide for privacy. Do not expose the client unnecessarily.
_____	_____	_____	4. Shake down the thermometer to 96°F (35.5°C).
_____	_____	_____	5. Position client on left side, Sims' position. Cover the client with a sheet or blanket and remove the client's clothing from the rectal area of the body.
_____	_____	_____	6. Lubricate the bulb tip of the thermometer with a water-soluble jelly and a tissue. This makes insertion easier and more comfortable.
_____	_____	_____	7. Fold back the sheet or blanket to expose the client's buttocks. Raise top buttock with your hand and, with the other hand, gently insert bulb end of thermometer into the client's rectum about 1 to 1½ inches.
_____	_____	_____	8. Redrape the client and hold the thermometer in place for 3 to 5 minutes. **Caution:** Do not let go of the rectal thermometer.
_____	_____	_____	9. Remove the thermometer; wipe it from stem to bulb end (clean to dirty).
_____	_____	_____	10. Discard contaminated tissue.

Practice	Satisfactory	Unsatisfactory	Procedural Steps
_____	_____	_____	11. Read the thermometer and record the temperature. Record the time and place the letter *R* (rectal) beside the temperature reading.
_____	_____	_____	12. Return the client to a comfortable position.
_____	_____	_____	13. Clean the thermometer using soap and cold water or alcohol. Rinse it thoroughly. Store properly.
_____	_____	_____	14. Remove gloves and wash your hands thoroughly after the procedure.

PROCEDURE 51:   TAKING AN AXILLARY TEMPERATURE

All items must be successfully completed in this skill. The practice column is for student/partner use. The instructor will check, date, and initial the other two columns.

Practice	Satisfactory	Unsatisfactory	Procedural Steps
_____	_____	_____	1. Wash your hands before beginning the procedure.
_____	_____	_____	2. Rinse the thermometer in cold water and wipe it dry with a tissue.
_____	_____	_____	3. Shake down the thermometer so the mercury is below 96°F (35.6°C).
_____	_____	_____	4. Dry the client's armpit with a tissue.
_____	_____	_____	5. Place the thermometer in the center of the client's axilla (armpit) with the bulb end toward the client's head. This position rests the bulb end against the blood vessel and a more accurate reading can be obtained.
_____	_____	_____	6. Position the client's arm close to the body and place the client's forearm over the client's chest. This position enables the arm to hold the thermometer in place.
_____	_____	_____	7. Leave the thermometer in place for 10 minutes.
_____	_____	_____	8. Remove the thermometer and wipe it clean of any perspiration.
_____	_____	_____	9. Read the temperature indicated on the thermometer. (A normal axillary temperature is 97.6°F.)
_____	_____	_____	10. Record the temperature. An axillary temperature is recorded with an *Ax* beside the number, e.g., 97.6°F Ax.
_____	_____	_____	11. Shake down the thermometer, clean it, and return it to its proper place.
_____	_____	_____	12. Wash your hands following the procedure.

PROCEDURE 52:   TAKING THE RADIAL AND APICAL PULSE

All items must be successfully completed in this skill. The practice column is for student/partner use. The instructor will check, date, and initial the other two columns.

Practice	*Satisfactory*	*Unsatisfactory*	*Procedural Steps*
			Determining Pulse Rate
_____	_____	_____	1. Gather the equipment needed: wrist watch with a second hand note pad and pen or pencil
_____	_____	_____	2. Wash your hands before beginning the procedure.
_____	_____	_____	3. Tell the client that you are going to check the pulse rate. Ask the client to help by remaining quiet and still while you are counting.
_____	_____	_____	4. Have the client sit in a comfortable chair or lie in bed with arms resting gently on the chest.
_____	_____	_____	5. Place the tips of your first two fingers on the pulse site. The radial pulse on the inner wrist is most often used. **Caution:** Do not use your thumb to feel the client's artery. Using the thumb can result in an inaccurate reading.
_____	_____	_____	6. Count the pulse beats for 1 full minute.
_____	_____	_____	7. Record the pulse rate, regularity, and strength. Also record the time the pulse was taken. If irregular, take apical for 1 minute and record apical pulse.
			Taking Apical Pulse
_____	_____	_____	1. Assemble equipment. stethoscope watch with second hand
_____	_____	_____	2. Tell client what you plan to do.
_____	_____	_____	3. Clean stethoscope earpieces and bell with disinfectant.
_____	_____	_____	4. Place stethoscope earpieces in your ears.

Practice	Satisfactory	Unsatisfactory		Procedural Steps
_____	_____	_____	5.	Place the stethoscope diaphragm or bell over the apex of the client's heart, 2 to 3 inches to the left of the breastbone, below the left nipple.
_____	_____	_____	6.	Listen carefully for the heart beat. It will sound like "lub-dub."
_____	_____	_____	7.	Count the louder sound for 1 complete minute.
_____	_____	_____	8.	Check radial pulse for 1 minute. The best way to obtain these numbers is to have an aide count the apical pulse. Another aide may take the radial pulse at the same time the apical pulse is being counted.
_____	_____	_____	9.	Compare the results and note the numbers on a pad.
_____	_____	_____	10.	Clean earpieces and bell or diaphragm of stethoscope with alcohol wipe
_____	_____	_____	11.	Document both pulse rates, i.e.,

apical pulse = A 100 @10:00 AM

radial pulse = R 92

Pulse deficit: 8 (100−92 = 8)

All items must be successfully completed in this skill. The practice column is for student/partner use. The instructor will check, date, and initial the other two columns.

Practice	Satisfactory	Unsatisfactory	Procedural Steps
_____	_____	_____	1. Gather equipment needed: wrist watch with a second hand note pad and pen or pencil
_____	_____	_____	2. After client's pulse has been taken, leave the fingers in position on the wrist. By doing this, the client is not aware that you are counting respirations.
_____	_____	_____	3. One rise and fall of the chest counts as one respiration. Count the number of respirations during a full 1-minute period.
_____	_____	_____	4. Note how deeply the client breathes. Also check the regularity of the rhythm pattern. Note the sound of the breathing.
_____	_____	_____	5. Record the number of respirations occuring in 1 minute. Record the character of the client's breathing.
_____	_____	_____	6. Report changes from the client's usual way of breathing. Report any difficulty in breathing to the supervisor at once.
_____	_____	_____	7. Wash your hands following the procedure.

PROCEDURE 54: TAKING A BLOOD PRESSURE

All items must be successfully completed in this skill. The practice column is for student/partner use. The instructor will check, date, and initial the other two columns.

Practice	Satisfactory	Unsatisfactory	Procedural Steps
_____	_____	_____	1. Gather equipment needed: sphygmomanometer stethoscope alcohol sponges or cotton balls
_____	_____	_____	2. Wash your hands before beginning the procedure.
_____	_____	_____	3. Explain to the client what you plan to do. Have the client sit or lie in a comfortable position with one arm extended at the same level as the heart. The palm should be upward. Arm should be in resting position. Locate brachial pulse.
_____	_____	_____	4. Pick up the stethoscope. Wipe the earpieces. Place the stethoscope around your neck.
_____	_____	_____	5. Pick up the cuff and wrap it securely around the client's arm, about 1 inch above the elbow. Fasten. (Some cuffs have a Velcro fastener; others have hooks at the end of the cuff.) The center of the rubber bladder should be directly over the brachial artery. If the cuff is marked with an arrow, place cuff so that the arrow points over the brachial artery.
_____	_____	_____	6. Attach the manometer (the dial gauge) to the top of the cuff so you can read it.
_____	_____	_____	7. Tighten the small round valve that is located along the side of the rubber bulb. (This valve controls the pumping you will do later.)
_____	_____	_____	8. With the tips of your fingers, locate the artery on the inside of the client's elbow. When you feel a throbbing beat, you have located the artery. Keep your fingers on the spot. Never use your thumb since it, too, has a pulse beat.

Practice	Satisfactory	Unsatisfactory		Procedural Steps
_____	_____	_____	9.	Place the round disk of the stethoscope over the artery you located on the client (slipping your fingers to hold it in place). With your other hand, insert the earpieces in your ear.
_____	_____	_____	10.	Take the rubber bulb in your hand. Look at the dial gauge while you pump air into the cuff by squeezing the bulb. Pump until the reading on the dial gauge is about 180 to 200.
_____	_____	_____	11.	Listen with the stethoscope placed in your ears and the disk over the artery. You should not hear any sound.
_____	_____	_____	12.	While listening, slowly release the air by opening the valve located beside the bulb, using the thumb and forefinger. (This will cause air to escape from the cuff and the reading on the manometer will drop.) You may have to tighten the bulb valve if the air escapes too fast.
_____	_____	_____	13.	Listen carefully. When the first sound is heard, remember the number seen on the dial gauge. This is the systolic pressure.
_____	_____	_____	14.	Watch the dial continue to fall as the air escapes. When the thumping sound becomes a muffled sound, remember the number. This is the diastolic pressure.
_____	_____	_____	15.	Release the remainder of the air from the cuff and remove it, leaving the valve open.
_____	_____	_____	16.	Record the two readings. Blood pressure reading is written as a fraction with the systolic (top) listed first and the diastolic (bottom) written under the line; for example, BP $\frac{120 \text{ (systolic pressure)}}{80 \text{ (diastolic pressure)}}$.
_____	_____	_____	17.	**Caution:** Be careful not to pump the pressure too high. Remember that the pressure of the cuff can cause the client discomfort so it is important to release the air and work quickly when taking the blood pressure. If it is necessary to repeat the procedure, wait a few minutes before inflating the cuff; this allows the circulation to return to normal.

Practice	Satisfactory	Unsatisfactory		Procedural Steps
_____	_____	_____	18.	If you are unsuccessful in obtaining a blood pressure reading after three attempts, move to the client's other arm and try again, repeating the same procedure. (A reading taken after three attempts would probably be inaccurate and the client would become uncomfortable.) Never guess. If a blood pressure is hard to take or you are not sure, tell the nurse. Record reading.
_____	_____	_____	19.	Wash your hands following the procedure.

Precautions

- If you are taking the blood pressure of a stroke client, use the unaffected arm only.

- If your client is having home dialysis (as part of a kidney treatment), or is receiving intravenous (IV) fluids, take the blood pressure on the unaffected arm.

- Do not inflate cuff unnecessarily high.

PROCEDURE 55:   MEASURING WEIGHT AND HEIGHT

All items must be successfully completed in this skill. The practice column is for student/partner use. The instructor will check, date, and initial the other two columns.

Practice	*Satisfactory*	*Unsatisfactory*	*Procedural Steps*
			Weight
_____	_____	_____	1. Client should be weighed at the same time of day.
_____	_____	_____	2. Client should be wearing the same amount of clothing each time.
_____	_____	_____	3. Scale should be checked to see if it is balanced correctly.
_____	_____	_____	4. Record and document weight.
			Height
_____	_____	_____	1. Have client positioned in bed flat on his back with arms and legs straight.
_____	_____	_____	2. Make a small pencil mark at the top of the client's head on the sheet.
_____	_____	_____	3. Make a second pencil mark even with the feet.
_____	_____	_____	4. Using the tape measure, measure the distance between the two marks.
_____	_____	_____	5. Record the height on the paper and record in client's record.
_____	_____	_____	6. If client can stand, have the client stand with his back to the wall. Mark the wall with a small pencil mark on top of client's head. Client is not to wear shoes.
_____	_____	_____	7. Measure from floor to small pencil mark with tape measure.
_____	_____	_____	8. Record on paper and then on client's chart.

PROCEDURE 56:   APPLYING AN ICE BAG, CAP, OR COLLAR

All items must be successfully completed in this skill. The practice column is for student/partner use. The instructor will check, date, and initial the other two columns.

Practice	*Satisfactory*	*Unsatisfactory*	*Procedural Steps*
_____	_____	_____	1. Wash your hands before beginning the procedure.
_____	_____	_____	2. Fill an ice bag, cap, or collar with ice cubes or crushed ice. Use a spoon to transfer the ice. Fill the container half full so that its weight will not be uncomfortable for the client.
_____	_____	_____	3. Place the bag on a flat surface with the top in place but not tightened. Hold the neck of the bag upright. Gently press the bag from the bottom to the opening in order to expel the air.
_____	_____	_____	4. Secure lid firmly and wipe dry with paper towels. Periodically test for leakage.
_____	_____	_____	5. Wrap ice bag in towel or soft cloth. Covering it protects the client's skin from direct contact. A disposable cold pack can also be used.
_____	_____	_____	6. Apply to affected body area. Make sure that any metal parts face away from the skin. Place an extra towel around the bag if the skin appears sensitive to the cold.
_____	_____	_____	7. Check the client's skin every 5 minutes. Look for signs of redness, whiteness, or cyanosis (blue color). If these signs appear, call the supervisor for instructions.
_____	_____	_____	8. If ice melts, replace with fresh ice and continue treatment.
_____	_____	_____	9. Remove ice bag after 20 minutes.
_____	_____	_____	10. Empty bag, allow it to dry. Store it properly.
_____	_____	_____	11. Return client to a comfortable position.
_____	_____	_____	12. Wash your hands following the procedure.

PROCEDURE 57: APPLYING A K-PAD—MOIST OR DRY

All items must be successfully completed in this skill. The practice column is for student/partner use. The instructor will check, date, and initial the other two columns.

Practice	Satisfactory	Unsatisfactory	Procedural Steps
_____	_____	_____	1. Assemble supplies: K-Pad and control unit distilled water cover for pad (a pillow case can be used) warm wet towel (if moist application) large plastic bag—optional
_____	_____	_____	2. Wash your hands.
_____	_____	_____	3. Tell client what you plan to do.
_____	_____	_____	4. Place the control unit close to the client on a stand.
_____	_____	_____	5. Remove the cover and fill the unit with distilled water to the fill line.
_____	_____	_____	6. Screw the cover in place and loosen it one-quarter turn.
_____	_____	_____	7. The temperature, usually 95°F to 100°F, is set by a key. Turn unit on and let the pad warm up a few minutes.
_____	_____	_____	8. Cover pad and place it on the client. Secure the pad if necessary with tape. Never use pins. Be sure that the tubing is coiled on the bed or chair to facilitate the flow of water inside the pad. Do not let the tubing hang down below the chair or bed.
_____	_____	_____	9. If the application is to be a moist application, warm a towel under hot water and wring out excess water. Wrap plastic bag and take to client. Apply moist towel, then K-pad and if necessary wrap with plastic bag or linen protector to keep area around the moist application dry.
_____	_____	_____	10. Note time of application. Follow orders on length of time the treatment should last.
_____	_____	_____	11. Check the control unit periodically. Refill as needed.
_____	_____	_____	12. Wash hands.
_____	_____	_____	13. Document completion of the procedure, your observations, and client's reaction.

PROCEDURE 58: PERFORMING A WARM FOOT SOAK

All items must be successfully completed in this skill. The practice column is for student/partner use. The instructor will check, date, and initial the other two columns.

Practice	Satisfactory	Unsatisfactory	Procedural Steps
_____	_____	_____	1. Assemble equipment: large basin—plastic oblong dishpan warm water—100° to 110°F large plastic garbage bag or sheet of plastic small thin blanket 2 towels
_____	_____	_____	2. Wash hands and apply gloves.
_____	_____	_____	3. Tell client what you plan to do.
_____	_____	_____	4. Have client sit in comfortable chair if possible.
_____	_____	_____	5. Place plastic bag on floor and place basin of water on top of plastic covering.
_____	_____	_____	6. Remove client's shoes and socks and slowly place client's feet in basin of warm water. Be sure to follow any special instructions for special soaps or solutions that might be ordered.
_____	_____	_____	7. Place thin blanket over the client's legs and feet.
_____	_____	_____	8. Replenish water as necessary to maintain proper temperature.
_____	_____	_____	9. Discontinue treatment in 20 to 30 minutes.
_____	_____	_____	10. Remove feet from basin and pat dry. Be sure to dry well in between toes. When feet are dry, massage lotion on both feet. Put shoes and socks on client's feet.
_____	_____	_____	11. Clean up equipment and return to storage area.
_____	_____	_____	12. Wash hands.
_____	_____	_____	13. Document completion of procedure, your observations, and client's reaction.

PROCEDURE 59:   GIVING A COMMERCIAL ENEMA

All items must be successfully completed in this skill. The practice column is for student/partner use. The instructor will check, date, and initial the other two columns.

Practice	Satisfactory	Unsatisfactory		Procedural Steps
_____	_____	_____	1.	Assemble supplies:
				gloves
				commercial prepackaged enema
				protective pad
				bedpan (if client is bedridden)
				toilet paper
				lubrication jelly
_____	_____	_____	2.	Wash hands and put on gloves.
_____	_____	_____	3.	Tell client what you plan to do.
_____	_____	_____	4.	Provide for the client's comfort and privacy.
_____	_____	_____	5.	Have client turn to left side. Turn covers back to expose only the buttocks.
_____	_____	_____	6.	Remove cover on tip of enema. Apply extra lubricant to tip to ensure easy insertion.
_____	_____	_____	7.	Place protective pad underneath the client's buttocks.
_____	_____	_____	8.	Separate the buttocks and insert tip into rectum for at least 3 inches. Tell client to take a deep breath and hold the solution as long as possible. Slowly squeeze the flexible plastic tube. This forces the solution to flow evenly into the rectum.
_____	_____	_____	9.	Remove enema tip while holding the client's buttocks together.
_____	_____	_____	10.	Position client on bedpan, commode, or toilet.
_____	_____	_____	11.	After client has expelled feces and enema solution, assist the client in cleaning area around anus and buttocks.
_____	_____	_____	12.	Return client to comfortable position. It may be necessary to leave the protective pad in place until the effects of the enema are complete.

Practice	Satisfactory	Unsatisfactory		Procedural Steps
_____	_____	_____	13.	Remove gloves and wash hands.
_____	_____	_____	14.	Record results of enema—color, amount, consistency—10:00 AM, Fleet's enema given, good results—large, brown, formed stool.

PROCEDURE 60:   GIVING A RECTAL SUPPOSITORY

All items must be successfully completed in this skill. The practice column is for student/partner use. The instructor will check, date, and initial the other two columns.

Practice	Satisfactory	Unsatisfactory		Procedural Steps
_____	_____	_____	1.	Assemble supplies:
				rectal suppository
				gloves
				lubricant
				protective pad or paper towels
_____	_____	_____	2.	Wash hands and apply gloves.
_____	_____	_____	3.	Tell client what you plan to do.
_____	_____	_____	4.	Open foil-wrapped suppository. Turn client to one side.
_____	_____	_____	5.	Lubricate gloved finger and insert suppository into rectum. Push the suppository along the lining of the rectum with your index finger as far as your finger allows. Be careful not to insert suppository into the feces. The suppository needs to be next to the lining of the colon for it to be effective.
_____	_____	_____	6.	After 10 minutes has passed, assist the client to the toilet or commode.
_____	_____	_____	7.	After client has had a bowel movement, assist client back to bed or chair.
_____	_____	_____	8.	Observe results of elimination.
_____	_____	_____	9.	Remove gloves and wash hands.
_____	_____	_____	10.	Record results. It is important to note color, consistency, and amount.

PROCEDURE 61: TRAINING AND RETRAINING BOWELS

All items must be successfully completed in this skill. The practice column is for student/partner use. The instructor will check, date, and initial the other two columns.

Practice	*Satisfactory*	*Unsatisfactory*	*Procedural Steps*
_____	_____	_____	1. The health care team assesses prior habits of a client. If client always had a bowel movement early in the morning, this would be important to know in planning the client's retraining program.
_____	_____	_____	2. A plan is designed and implemented. Important elements of the plan are: • high intake of fiber foods • adequate intake of liquids • regular exercise • toileting client at regular intervals • praise by aide of slightest progress of client • less reliance on laxatives and enemas • privacy for client for bowel movements
_____	_____	_____	3. Follow bowel retraining program developed by the health care team. If plan does appear to be working, note success of program. If plan does not work, report. It is also important to give some suggestions to the health care team of possible solutions for retraining of the client.

PROCEDURE 62: APPLYING ADULT BRIEFS

All items must be successfully completed in this skill. The practice column is for student/partner use. The instructor will check, date, and initial the other two columns.

Practice	Satisfactory	Unsatisfactory		Procedural Steps
_____	_____	_____	1.	Wash hands
_____	_____	_____	2.	Gather equipment:
				undergarments
				proper type and size of brief needed (follow the plan of care)
				gloves as needed
_____	_____	_____	3.	Provide privacy for the client.
_____	_____	_____	4.	Apply briefs (Note: this may be done while the client is in bed or when the client is standing).
_____	_____	_____	5.	Follow directions for the brief itself if necessary (some have pull-apart tabs or snaps).
_____	_____	_____	6.	Check with the client to see that the brief fits *and* feels comfortable.
_____	_____	_____	7.	Check client frequently.
_____	_____	_____	8.	Wash hands.
_____	_____	_____	9.	Document results.

PROCEDURE 63: COLLECTING A STOOL SPECIMEN

All items must be successfully completed in this skill. The practice column is for student/partner use. The instructor will check, date, and initial the other two columns.

Practice	*Satisfactory*	*Unsatisfactory*	*Procedural Steps*
_____	_____	_____	1. Assemble needed supplies: gloves bedpan specimen container or hemoccult slide packet with label completed
_____	_____	_____	2. Inform client of need for specimen.
_____	_____	_____	3. After client has defecated in bedpan, apply gloves and with wood applicator remove stool. If specimen is to be collected in specimen container, place small amount (approximately 1 tablespoon) of stool in container. If the test is for occult blood or guaiac, place small amount of stool on hemoccult blood card.
_____	_____	_____	4. Place specimen in proper storage place. Be sure the specimen is sent to laboratory as directed by your supervisor.
_____	_____	_____	5. Remove gloves and wash hands.
_____	_____	_____	6. Document stool specimen collection.

PROCEDURE 64: APPLYING UNSTERILE DRESSING AND OINTMENT TO UNBROKEN SKIN

All items must be successfully completed in this skill. The practice column is for student/partner use. The instructor will check, date, and initial the other two columns.

Practice	Satisfactory	Unsatisfactory	Procedural Steps
_____	_____	_____	1. Assemble supplies: two or more 4 × 4 gauze pads prepackaged gloves over-the-counter ointment (if ordered) receptacle for wastes, i.e., plastic bag tape and scissors
_____	_____	_____	2. Wash your hands and apply gloves.
_____	_____	_____	3. Tell client what you plan to do.
_____	_____	_____	4. Position client so area with dressing is accessible while maintaining client comfort.
_____	_____	_____	5. Remove old dressing. If the dressing does not lift off easily, pour hydrogen peroxide over it to loosen it. Discard used dressing in open waste receptacle (plastic bag). Note color, amount of drainage, and condition of surrounding skin.
_____	_____	_____	6. Open the package of gauze pads without touching the pads. Be careful not to have dressing touch bed linens or client's clothing. Cut tape. Apply ointment if ordered. Apply dressing. Do not touch center of dressing. Hold all dressings on the corners only. Apply tape correctly.
_____	_____	_____	7. Position client comfortably.
_____	_____	_____	8. Discard wastes and return supplies to storage. Be sure to follow universal precautions throughout this procedure.
_____	_____	_____	9. Remove gloves and wash hands.
_____	_____	_____	10. Record observations of the wound and skin condition. Report signs of redness, swelling, heat, foul odor, or amount of drainage. Document dressing was changed. In addition, report client complaints of pain around the wound.

Practice	Satisfactory	Unsatisfactory	Procedural Steps
			Topical Applications to Unbroken Skin
_____	_____	_____	1. Obtain correct topical medication. Check label of medication with nursing care plan.
_____	_____	_____	2. Position client so area is accessible, while maintaining client comfort.
_____	_____	_____	3. Wash hands and apply gloves.
_____	_____	_____	4. Apply medication in a thin layer to affected area only. Note color and appearance of skin.
_____	_____	_____	5. Remove gloves and reposition client.
_____	_____	_____	6. Wash hands.
_____	_____	_____	7. Return medication to correct storage area.
_____	_____	_____	8. Chart treatment and appearance of skin.

PROCEDURE 65:   CARING FOR CASTS

All items must be successfully completed in this skill. The practice column is for student/partner use. The instructor will check, date, and initial the other two columns.

Practice	Satisfactory	Unsatisfactory	Procedural Steps
_____	_____	_____	1. Observe the new cast every 2 to 3 hours for the first 2 days and then 4 times daily.

    • Note the color of the skin at the farthest end of cast—normal pink, warm to touch, and movable toes or fingers.

    • Look for edema at both ends of the cast; report and record this information.

    • Observe for response to touch (that is the response of the nerves to stimulation); report and record this information.

Practice	Satisfactory	Unsatisfactory	Procedural Steps
_____	_____	_____	2. Observe the cast daily for roughness around the edges. This may cause skin irritation and may be filed or covered with soft padding. These rough edges can be covered with plain white tape. This is called petaling and can be done by the nurse.
_____	_____	_____	3. Observe the cast itself, noting any redness that may indicate bleeding or drainage from under the cast. Circle the area with a magic marker, noting the date and time that you first notice the marking. Also note any unusual odor. Record and report immediately.
_____	_____	_____	4. Observe the cast constantly for any cracks. Cracks are unsafe and you should notify your nurse supervisor of the crack. You must state the exact location and length of the crack as well as the depth of it.
_____	_____	_____	5. When the cast is near the perineal area, protect it from moisture. Ask your case manager for special instruction on what waterproof or protective device to use. Protect the cast and skin by preventing any dirt, sand, or small articles from getting inside the cast, which could cause an infection under the cast. Note that plaster of paris cast tends to crumble and become soft when moist; therefore, this type of cast must always be kept dry.

Practice	Satisfactory	Unsatisfactory	
			Procedural Steps
_____	_____	_____	6. Ask the client if he/she has pain in any particular area under the cast. This may indicate a pressure point and skin break-down under the cast. Note this area. Report and record immediately. Be sure to position your client correctly.

Safety for Client with a Cast

Practice	Satisfactory	Unsatisfactory	
_____	_____	_____	1. Check the house for throw rugs or objects on the floor. Remove any hazard that may cause the client to fall. Remind client to leave a night-light on to prevent a fall in the middle of the night.
_____	_____	_____	2. Remember that at first the client may not have a good sense of balance and may be unsteady in walking. Arrange the furniture so that the client may hold on to furniture or handrails while walking.
_____	_____	_____	3. Assist the client in making changes in eating, dressing, writing, toileting, and walking.
_____	_____	_____	4. Ask the case manager for specific orders for passive range of motion exercises. A physical therapist or occupational therapist may come to assist the client with specific exercises. A home health aide may not perform these exercises without orders and direct supervision.
_____	_____	_____	5. Determine the composition of the cast by asking the case manager. Plaster of paris casts take at least 24 hours to dry, while polyester or fiberglass casting tape takes 5 to 15 minutes to dry. Be sure you do not touch the wet cast because fingers may leave dents in the cast. Do not allow cast to dry on hard surface, as this will flatten the cast. Do place entire new cast on pillows and expose to air. Do not allow client to put anything between the cast and the skin if the skin under the cast starts to itch. If itching becomes unbearable, air can be blown in by use of a hair dryer, if the nurse supervisor gives you permission to do this. When positioning a client with an extremity cast, elevate the cast on pillows. Generally it is not allowable to have the client lie on the injured side. Instruct the client to wiggle toes or fingers frequently on cast extremity. Do not cover cast extremity because air needs to be allowed to circulate inside the cast.

PROCEDURE 66:   ASSISTING WITH CHANGING AN OSTOMY BAG

All items must be successfully completed in this skill. The practice column is for student/partner use. The instructor will check, date, and initial the other two columns.

Practice	Satisfactory	Unsatisfactory	Procedural Steps
_____	_____	_____	1. Assemble supplies: basin of warm water and soap clean ostomy bag double bags gloves skin ointment (if ordered) toilet tissue
_____	_____	_____	2. Wash your hands and apply gloves.
_____	_____	_____	3. Tell client what you plan to do.
_____	_____	_____	4. Gently remove soiled colostomy bag from the stoma. Place in double-bagged receptacle. In a few instances, the colostomy bag can be washed and reused.
_____	_____	_____	5. If there is stool on the skin remove with toilet tissue. Wash area around the stoma with mild soap and water. Pat the area dry. Occasionally a special substance may be applied to assist the new colostomy bag to adhere better.
_____	_____	_____	6. Apply ointment if ordered. Observe area around the stoma for redness or open areas.
_____	_____	_____	7. Apply client's pouch. • If one-piece pouch or bag is being used, remove self-stick backing from new ostomy appliance. Press the new bag to the area around the stoma, being sure to seal tightly. • If two-piece pouch is being used, be sure to cut opening to the correct size. (A few bags are premeasured and this step is not necessary.) Remove adhesive backing on face plate. Firmly apply face plate to client's skin around stoma, working from the stoma outward. Then apply the bag to this face plate. Let your client assist you as much as possible. Be sure to follow any special manufacturer's instruction in application of appliance.

Practice	Satisfactory	Unsatisfactory		Procedural Steps
_____	_____	_____	8.	Assist the client to connect belt to appliance, if client is using this type of appliance.
_____	_____	_____	9.	Remove wastes. Observe stool for color, amount, and consistency. If necessary spray the room with deodorizer.
_____	_____	_____	10.	Remove gloves and wash hands.
_____	_____	_____	11.	Document procedure and time, your observations, and client's reaction.

All items must be successfully completed in this skill. The practice column is for student/partner use. The instructor will check, date, and initial the other two columns.

Practice	*Satisfactory*	*Unsatisfactory*	*Procedural Steps*
_____	_____	_____	1. Check the meter of the oxygen tank or reservoir. If low, check to see if there is a spare tank. If there is not a spare tank, call for a replacement.
_____	_____	_____	2. Wash your hands before beginning the procedure.
_____	_____	_____	3. Check to see if the client's oxygen mask or cannula is placed properly. The straps on the cannula should be secure but not too tight. Check top of ears for signs of irritation. Check for signs of irritation where the prongs touch the client's nose. Be sure both prongs are in the client's nose. If a mask is being used, check to see whether the mask is over both nose and mouth. If inside of mask is wet, remove and dry inside.
_____	_____	_____	4. Check the gauge to see if the oxygen is being given at correct amount of liter flow. (Oxygen therapy is delivered in liters.) The client's care plan should state the liter flow to be administered to that client. Follow any special instructions that the respiratory therapist may prescribe.
_____	_____	_____	5. Check the client position. If in bed, elevate the head with three pillows to assist the client in breathing.
_____	_____	_____	6. Check to see if there is an adequate water supply for the humidifier. If you need to refill the humidifier, it is best to use distilled water. Humidification means adding moisture to oxygen. Oxygen is dry and can be irritating if used alone. Use of a humidifier with oxygen therapy is optional; some individuals do not require it. The respiratory therapist will instruct you on proper procedure on how to refill the humidifier on the oxygen tank your client has.

Practice	*Satisfactory*	*Unsatisfactory*		*Procedural Steps*
_____	_____	_____	7.	Do frequent mouth care for clients receiving oxygen therapy. Client's mouth can become dry and have an unpleasant taste. Apply lubricant to lips, if permitted, if they become dry.
_____	_____	_____	8.	Check that all safety precautions are being observed.

- Do not smoke in room where client is receiving oxygen. Post "No Smoking" sign, if necessary, to warn visitors not to smoke.

- Do not use matches, candles, or open flames where oxygen is used or stored.

- Do not use electrical appliances during oxygen therapy. Avoid sparks. If you need to shave the client, turn off the oxygen while using the electric razor.

- Avoid use of woolen blankets, which may create static electricity sparks.

_____	_____	_____	9.	Wash your hands.
_____	_____	_____	10.	Document the liter flow and the device being used, your observations, and client's reaction.

PROCEDURE 68: ASSISTING WITH COUGH AND DEEP BREATHING EXERCISES

All items must be successfully completed in this skill. The practice column is for student/partner use. The instructor will check, date, and initial the other two columns.

Practice	Satisfactory	Unsatisfactory	Procedural Steps
_____	_____	_____	1. Wash your hands.
_____	_____	_____	2. Tell client what you plan to do and ask for cooperation.
_____	_____	_____	3. Assemble equipment needed: gloves—optional pillow case-covered pillow tissues small basin or receptacle
_____	_____	_____	4. Have client sit up if possible.
_____	_____	_____	5. Have client place hands on either side of rib cage or operative site. A pillow over operative site may be used to support incision during the breathing exercises.
_____	_____	_____	6. Ask client to take as deep a breath through the nose as possible and hold it for 5 to 7 seconds and then exhale slowly through pursed lips.
_____	_____	_____	7. Repeat this exercise about five times unless the client is too tired.
_____	_____	_____	8. Give client tissues and instruct client to take a deep breath and cough forcefully twice with mouth open. Collect any secretions that are brought up in tissues. Protect yourself from secretions and droplets.
_____	_____	_____	9. Put on gloves if you will be touching or handling the tissues.
_____	_____	_____	10. Dispose of tissues in plastic bag and assist client to comfortable position.
_____	_____	_____	11. Remove gloves and wash hands.
_____	_____	_____	12. Document procedure completed, your observations, and client's reaction.

PROCEDURE 69: ASSISTING WITH BREAST-FEEDING AND BREAST CARE

All items must be successfully completed in this skill. The practice column is for student/partner use. The instructor will check, date, and initial the other two columns.

Practice	Satisfactory	Unsatisfactory	Procedural Steps
_____	_____	_____	1. Provide supplies: mild soap warm water in basin clean washcloth and towel clean nursing bra (or well-fitting support bra) nursing pads cotton balls rinse water in basin (at feeding time) clock or watch to time nursing period
_____	_____	_____	2. Wash your hands thoroughly before beginning the procedure.
_____	_____	_____	3. Help the mother to wash her hands before handling the breasts.
_____	_____	_____	4. Help the mother open the front of her dress or shirt top, if needed. Have mother wash nipples in warm water and mild soap using a circular motion, washing from the nipple outward. Rinse and dry the breasts thoroughly. (La Leche League suggests that washing the nipple before each feeding can lead to drying and cracking and should be avoided. Consult your physician.)
_____	_____	_____	5. Have mother sit in comfortable position in a rocking chair with armrest and footstool to support the feet. If mother is still on bed rest, help her lie on one side.
_____	_____	_____	6. Change infant's diaper; wash your hands thoroughly after the diaper change.
_____	_____	_____	7. Bring child to mother. Make sure infant's nose is not pressed against the mother's breast. The nostrils must be free so the infant can breathe as it nurses. Follow procedure as taught in hospital unless unsuccessful.

Practice	Satisfactory	Unsatisfactory		Procedural Steps
_____	_____	_____	8.	The nursing period is gradually built up from just a few minutes to a maximum of 20 minutes. Some mothers prefer to let baby nurse at both breasts (one at a time) during one feeding period. Others will feed the infant only at one breast for each 20-minute feeding period. They alternate breasts at different feedings.
_____	_____	_____	9.	To remove the baby's mouth from the breast, have mother press on two sides of nipple to release the suction.
_____	_____	_____	10.	At the end of the feeding period, return baby to crib. Make sure the baby has been burped before it is laid down. Change diaper if necessary.
_____	_____	_____	11.	Wash your hands before continuing with the procedure.
_____	_____	_____	12.	Help the mother with her bra, putting fresh nursing pads over the nipples to absorb any leakage. If nipples are sore or cracked, have the mother contact the nurse. An ointment or medication may be prescribed. Report these problems to the case manager.
_____	_____	_____	13.	Return supplies to storage.
_____	_____	_____	14.	Wash your hands following the procedure.

PROCEDURE 70:   GIVING THE INFANT A SPONGE BATH

All items must be successfully completed in this skill. The practice column is for student/partner use. The instructor will check, date, and initial the other two columns.

Practice	Satisfactory	Unsatisfactory		Procedural Steps
_____	_____	_____	1.	Bring needed supplies to kitchen table or baby's bath table:
				warm water in basin (test temperature)
				towel and washcloth
				bath sheets
				diapers (cloth or disposable paper)
				bath oil
				baby lotion
				baby shampoo
				change of clothing (undershirt, gown, etc.)
				mild soap
_____	_____	_____	2.	Wash your hands thoroughly before beginning the procedure.
_____	_____	_____	3.	Lower siderail of crib. Keep the rail raised to its highest position whenever infant is in crib. Bring infant to bathing area.
_____	_____	_____	4.	Place infant on bath sheet and undress. Drop soiled diaper into diaper pail. Close diaper pins and keep out of baby's reach. **Caution:** NEVER leave baby unattended while it is on the bath table.
_____	_____	_____	5.	Place infant in bath basin. Wash the infant's face with warm water only. Do not use soap on the face. Pat face dry. Make sure ears are carefully dried. Wash neck and pat dry. Rub in small amount of lotion around creases in baby's neck.
_____	_____	_____	6.	Gently apply a small amount of soap over baby's head and lather well to remove crust. Rinse soap away by holding head over basin as you repeatedly wipe head with wet washcloth. Keep soap out of infant's eyes. If soap is left on scalp, it will cause scales to crust and collect. Dry scalp carefully. Rub on baby oil.
_____	_____	_____	7.	Lather your hands and apply soap to the infant's hands, arms, and chest. Rinse completely with washcloth.

Practice	Satisfactory	Unsatisfactory		Procedural Steps
_____	_____	_____	8.	Apply soap to abdomen and legs and lather well. Rinse with washcloth.
_____	_____	_____	9.	Turn infant on the stomach and lather the infant's back; rinse and dry.
_____	_____	_____	10.	Wash, rinse, and dry genital (perineal) area last. Uncircumcised males should have the foreskin pushed back gently and the area washed with water only. Wash the penis and folds of the scrotum. Dry infant.
_____	_____	_____	11.	Dress infant. Return to crib or playpen.
_____	_____	_____	12.	Return supplies to storage. Clean up area where bath was given.
_____	_____	_____	13.	Wash your hands following the procedure.

PROCEDURE 71:   BOTTLE-FEEDING THE INFANT

All items must be successfully completed in this skill. The practice column is for student/partner use. The instructor will check, date, and initial the other two columns.

Practice	Satisfactory	Unsatisfactory		Procedural Steps
_____	_____	_____	1.	Wash your hands before beginning the procedure.
_____	_____	_____	2.	Prepare formula as directed. Pour into baby bottle.
_____	_____	_____	3.	Change infant's diaper, if necessary, so infant will be comfortable, clean, and dry while eating. Wrap infant loosely in a clean receiving blanket. Leave infant in crib with side rails up.
_____	_____	_____	4.	Wash your hands.
_____	_____	_____	5.	Bring warm bottle to table next to a comfortable rocker or armchair.
_____	_____	_____	6.	Support infant's head and back when picking it up from the crib. Sit comfortably in chair, holding child securely in a comfortable position for taking nipple; start to feed the infant. Do not prop bottle.
_____	_____	_____	7.	When infant has had 2 to 3 ounces, either sit the infant upright on your lap and gently pat back or hold the infant over your shoulder and pat its back until the infant burps.
_____	_____	_____	8.	Continue feeding and burping until infant is finished or shows no interest in eating. Do not force infant to take more than it wants.
_____	_____	_____	9.	When the baby is finished, burp it once more then place it in the crib lying it on its side or stomach. DO NOT PLACE THE INFANT ON BACK. If infant should regurgitate, there would be a possibility of causing serious hazard.
_____	_____	_____	10.	Wash your hands following the procedure. **Caution:** Do not put infant to bed with bottle and do not prop bottle. Spend as much time as you can with the infant and interact with the infant.